LIVING WELL
ON THE ROAD

LIVING WELL ON THE ROAD

HEALTH AND WELLNESS FOR TRAVELERS

LINDEN SCHAFFER

ROWMAN & LITTLEFIELD
Lanham • Boulder • New York • London

Published by Rowman & Littlefield
A wholly owned subsidiary of The Rowman & Littlefield Publishing Group, Inc.
4501 Forbes Boulevard, Suite 200, Lanham, Maryland 20706
www.rowman.com

Unit A, Whitacre Mews, 26-34 Stannary Street, London SE11 4AB

Distributed by NATIONAL BOOK NETWORK

British Library Cataloguing in Publication Information Available

Library of Congress Cataloging-in-Publication Data Available

ISBN 978-1-4422-6210-2 (pbk. : alk. paper)
ISBN 978-1-4422-6211-9 (electronic)

♾™ The paper used in this publication meets the minimum requirements of American National Standard for Information Sciences—Permanence of Paper for Printed Library Materials, ANSI/NISO Z39.48-1992.
Printed in the United States of America

CONTENTS

FOREWORD

People travel for all sorts of reasons—to see the world, to rest, to escape, to boast, to gain another perspective—but I think the reason people *continue* to travel, the reason they are willing to suffer the indignities of the road—the headaches, the inconveniences, and the hassles—is because in some real way travel brings people home to themselves. Rarely have I felt that paradoxical pleasure of being more comfortable in my skin than when I am in some far-flung locale, surrounded by unfamiliar sights, sounds, and smells. Perhaps that feeling of "at homeness" so far from home is one definition of a traveler.

If so, then Linden Schaffer falls into the category of a true traveler. I met Linden a number of years ago, fresh upon her return from several months in Asia. Flush with the energy of an expansive session of travel, she spoke of how she longed to create experiences for people—journeys of a mind-body-spirit merging that would serve the whole traveler. I watched over the next several years as she did just that—through Pravassa—creating itineraries that people could not only relax into but grow through.

Yet the real challenge of every traveler comes after the suit-case is unpacked. Exactly how do we bring those "best version of ourselves" feelings back, and carry them forward into our daily existence? By sharing her own story and knowledge gleaned through years of experience on the road, Linden has captured that know-how in these pages and offers it up for us. Imbued with her unique spirit of adventure and generosity, *Living Well On the Road* brings it all home.

Andrew McCarthy

If your body aches from the constant tension of stress; if your mouth waters from the mention of sugary junk food; if you have a complete lack of mental focus for more than 10 minutes at a time; if you skip exercising in the name of exhaustion and rely on more than one cup of caffeine to make it through the day; *this book is for you.* Replace the smartphone next to your bed with it and start your road to wellness—one that can only be designed and maintained by you. Once you gain an understanding of today's wellness environment and the tools available to help you both at home and on the road, any perceived barriers will be blown away as you create a personal path toward optimal health and happiness.

Warning: side effects may include increased energy, a stabilized mood, lowered stress levels, fewer colds, a sense of overall awesomeness, and a newly discovered real happiness and well-being.

INTRODUCTION

Practice Makes Perfect

Early on in my glamorous (and painfully fast-paced) fashion career, I realized something: the way I worked was turning me from a poised, intelligent human being into a tightly wound little ball of stress and tension. For 15 New York City rat race years, I conducted business all over the United States and Europe for multiple companies.

I spent a huge chunk of my life at a desk, having late night client dinners and hustling from airports to hotels to meetings and back again. During this time, work became a struggle instead of a joy. I ate whatever was in front of me and slept when I could. I was biting my nails and shopping to try to buy happiness. I had no energy to see family or friends. I came home from every conference, sales meeting, and business trip feeling more and more exhausted by the pace of my life. My health started to deteriorate. I felt like crap.

Make no mistake, I loved my high-stakes career, but I felt a primal need to take control over my well-being. Something clearly needed to change. One evening while sitting in my hotel room in Italy with tears rolling down my face, I decided I didn't want to feel like this any longer—this was my Aha! moment, and it changed everything.

Giving myself permission to take back control over my own self-care was my first step toward wellness, and it allowed me the opportunity to be open to creating easy solutions for my hectic schedule struggles. A day of back-to-back meetings that started in a sterile hotel room was depressing, which meant my wellness solution was to wake up 30 minutes early and spend time outdoors breathing in nature's fresh air. Standing on my feet in high heels for 12-hour days at a trade show abusing my body meant my wellness solution was to skip cocktail hour in favor of rolling out a yoga mat. A red-eye flight across time zones that wreaked havoc with my circadian rhythm was a losing battle, which meant my wellness solution was absolutely no meetings scheduled until after lunch so I could have time to work out and sit in the sauna, detoxing the physical and mental stress of travel before meeting clients.

Mind you, the changes were not always massive leaps, but often just simple alterations. They were things that did not happen all at once, but as baby steps that helped me build a solid foundation and then stack healthy behaviors on top of each other. Fresh fruit instead of a bagel for breakfast, breathing exercises on the subway instead of catching a few extra winks, client dinners at locally sourced restaurants ... with every tiny change, my wellness boosted tenfold. I was able to slowly start integrating these decisions into my daily routine, which allowed me to explore new and better ways to take care of myself. Suddenly, I felt better and took fewer sick days than I had in years. My confidence started to build and I felt comfortable standing up for my well-being, as I knew it also improved my productivity. Everyone took notice. My coworkers started begging me for the secret.

That's when it hit me: I am not special. What I uncovered for myself was not magic; I was merely listening to my body. Whether you work in an office, out of your home or have the hard responsibility of being a full-time parent or caregiver, we are all stressed. We all have limited time. We are all looking for something more than a digitally dependent, jet-lagged, fast-food, sugar-laden existence. You deserve a foolproof wellness plan that will meaningfully modify your lifestyle, help you stay healthy—physically, mentally, and socially—and allow you to stand up for your self-care, even when you feel you don't have time.

After years of contemplating my next career move, I realized wellness was where my true passion lay, and that my enthusiasm and "lived-in" results resonated with those around me.

I made the leap and left the fashion world to start Pravassa, the first wellness travel company, in hopes of helping others kickstart their health, happiness, and wellness lifestyle on the road, then supporting them in their journey once they returned home.

I spent a year studying for a wellness certification, and shortly after becoming a solopreneur—a solo entrepreneur single-handedly responsible for my start-up business—British Airways recognized Pravassa as a winner in its Face of Opportunity contest. As a pioneer at the forefront of the wellness travel movement, I have spoken at the *Los Angeles Times* and *New York Times* travel shows, completed a 10 episode wellness video series for *Livestrong.com*, and have participated in a leadership summit organized by the Global Wellness Institute. As the concept of healthy living and wellness travel gains worldwide recognition, tourism boards from Spain, India, and Colombia have hosted me in order to foster wellness opportunities outside of the United States.

As a leading expert in my field, I am a regular contributor to *The Huffington Post's* Lifestyle and Travel columns, to the largest online wellness community *mindbodygreen.com*, and to *SpaFinder Wellness 365*. In these columns, I write about everything from simple living-well tips to wellness travel advice and hot spot destinations. And Pravassa has been featured in *Condé Nast Traveler, the LA Times, the Chicago Tribune, Forbes, International Business Times*, and *New York Magazine* among others.

I decided to write this book because it is time for every busy, stressed-out person to advocate for his or her self-care. You deserve a complete approach to your personal well-being whether you spend most of your time in an office, traveling for work, or are a solopreneur like me. In this book, you will find personal stories, tips, and tricks, backed by scientific research and the latest health and wellness studies combined.

Why is finding a wellness balance so important? Because it increases productivity, refocuses attention, puts your health back on track, and helps you have feel-good experiences that release stress and tension from your body, mind, and social interactions. When you understand how to set yourself up for a wellness experience, you will not only feel better and notice significant change, but you will begin to make balanced choices for every aspect of your life and the lives of those around you.

A PEEK AT WHAT'S INSIDE

- An easy to understand wellness philosophy, which will be your key to defining and implementing wellness for you— at home, at work, and eventually on the road.
- The latest scientific data, studies, and surveys across multiple subsectors of wellness in pared-down, easy-to-understand language.
- Chapters titled "Get Rest," "Get Fit," "Get Zen," "Get Local," and "Get Food" will delve into real-life sustainable changes that lead to results.
- Interviews with today's leading experts in the fields of psychology, stress management, and integrative health— people on the forefront of creating wellness programs that have proven impact on personal health and wellness.
- Information on tracking results. In our technology-driven society, wearable tracking devices lead the charge in personal evidence-based results.
- Tips and tricks that will allow you to continue your wellness practices with flourishing results when you take with them with you on the road.
- Wellness checklists that will help you skip the trial-and-error phase of creating a new lifestyle routine and get you straight to better health.

Living Well on the Road **is the complete playbook for wellness that works seamlessly alongside your current lifestyle.**

1

ARE WE WELL?

Your job is making you fat. And sick. And stressed. I know, I've been there. For 15 years, I was an active participant in New York City's rat race. Up before dawn, out the door, I would be lulled back to sleep on the subway ride into my office and hit the ground running at Rockefeller Center. Diet Coke in one hand, whole wheat wrap in the other. Between answering phone calls and emails, I'd squeeze in 20 minutes to eat at my desk, only to look up past sunset and realize another 10 hours had passed. Back on the train, I'd leaf through a magazine or thumb at a smartphone game to numb my brain from the day. Then, waiting for take-out at my neighborhood Thai dive, I'd glance at my watch, sickened by how little time stood between scarfing down the paper bag's contents in front of an episode of *Lost* and bedtime. After five-and-a-half hours of sleep (if I was lucky), my alarm would sound and I'd start the vicious cycle over again.

Sound Familiar?

If so, you are one of many on the corporate ladder striving toward the top rungs of your career, family, and financial expectations without the supportive foundation needed for your well-being. Whatever you gain, however, is at the expense of your health, made worse by a laundry list of bad habits: lack of sleep, grueling schedules, unhealthy eating, and irregular exercise. Caught in a vicious cycle when it comes to managing our lives, these hefty barriers make any positive lifestyle or behavioral change seem near impossible.

In 1948, the World Health Organization defined wellness as "a state of complete physical, mental, and social well-being, not merely the absence of disease."[1] An article published in the 2014 *Journal of American Psychosomatic Medicine* concluded that men and women who experience high stress at work carry a higher risk of developing type 2 diabetes.[2] Aside from the typical genetic factors, excess weight gain and the inactivity of sitting for hours on end are contributing factors to manifesting the disease. Most of us are managing stress poorly; any healthy lifestyle changes necessary to reach our optimal health are reducing as we cling to ineffective coping mechanisms.

According to the 2012 Stress in America survey, the harmful coping mechanisms of overeating and drinking alcohol to combat stress are on a steady decline, down 9% and 5%, respectively.[3] While this might appear to be a step in the right direction, we have replaced these behaviors with other sedentary habits including binge-watching TV, listening to music, or reading a book. These coping mechanisms may offer short-term relief, but can exacerbate long-term physical issues and still leave us lying awake at night mindlessly reaching for unhealthy foods or dangerously skipping meals altogether. The long-term side effects of these fruitless tactics can manifest into irritability, anxiety, fatigue, mental exhaustion, loss of creativity, poor decision-making, chronic heartburn, depression, and lack of motivation. Not exactly positive steps in the direction of personal health and wellness.

AMERICA'S CURRENT HEALTHCARE SYSTEM

> *We do not have a "health care" system aimed at preventing illness, but rather a "disease management system" that overemphasizes drugs and surgery after the patient becomes ill.*[4]
>
> —Dr. Andrew Weil, director,
> Arizona Center for Integrative Medicine

The state of our national healthcare system is in flux. Not one program is comprehensive enough to predict, combat, and maintain personal well-being. The United States spends more on healthcare than any other country in the world, yet has the worst health outcomes when compared to all other developed nations.[5] In 2000, the World Health Organization ranked U.S. health outcomes in 37th place out of 191 countries. Ouch.

As a nation, we are not getting what we need or want from our current reactive disease management system, especially when it comes to behavioral health and stress-related illnesses. Of the 270 million people with health insurance in the United States, only 19% feel their healthcare coverage is providing what they need to maintain their health.[6] If you're grading, that's an F.

Chronic stress is the largest modern healthcare problem, and its overwhelming side effects continue to wreak havoc on our lives, playing a role in every one of America's top chronic illnesses. Cardiovascular disease, type 2 diabetes, ulcers, insomnia, and sexual dysfunction are all traceable to our lifestyle choices and therefore may be preventable. When left untreated, consistent high stress can develop into many other chronic conditions. Repeated exposure to high stress in the office or in your personal life may make you prone to bouts of anxiety, be the cause of your trouble sleeping, or leave you feeling unrested even after being in bed for 8 hours. You may burst into tears watching a TV commercial or yell at your children for a simple "kid" mistake. Add all this to muscle fatigue and physical body pain from prolonged sitting in front of your computer and electronic devices, which screws with concentration and weakens your immune system, and it's no wonder we open ourselves up to more serious health risks, all of which can lead to burnout or worse: the development of a major illness.

Wellness, as defined in today's medical community, is formal preventative care: immunizations and screenings for common diseases with attention paid to weight and unhealthy practices such as smoking, excessive drinking, and drug use. But today's general practitioner is not trained in prevention, unless your physician practices integrative medicine. Most physicians receive their bulk of training in medical schools and are trained to remove obstructions to your health once you already have them. By one doctor's own admission speaking at a wellness conference I attended, any of his additional on-the-job education typically arrives in the form of a young, pretty female pharmaceutical rep with free samples.

Think about it: we've been trained from a young age to go to the doctor only if we feel unwell or need a shot. Today if you are seeing your doctor for tests to find out what is wrong, you've most likely already missed the prevention boat. It is time to teach yourself how to manage your wellness so your next visit to the doctor can be to discuss how you are controlling your health, not your illness.

WORKPLACE WELLNESS

> Up until 2000, Corporate Wellness was a company nurse, health insurance and a benefits plan. Then corporations had a collective Aha! moment; it's not **Work** and **Life**, it's just life.[7]

> —Tevis Trower, founder of Balance Integration

Long hours and twenty-first-century lifestyle demands weigh heavily on our health and well-being. According to the Stress in American Study, people are struggling to manage the relationship between stress and health, with overall findings reporting that most working Americans believe their stress levels are higher than what is healthy.[8] When we are not given the tools or the support system to properly manage our stress levels, our stress increases, kicking off a downward spiral that can be hard to reverse.

In the office, employer-covered health insurance has been on a downward trend since 2008 according to the Gallup-Healthways Well-Being Index. With 57% of the working population currently covered,[9] this number continues to fall yearly, and future predictions do not appear to be getting brighter primarily due to the overall cost to employers. In a 10-year span from 2004 to 2014, the average annual health insurance premium has increased 69%,[10] with employee contribution climbing to an all-time high of 93%.[11] Of those still fortunate enough to be receiving employer-paid coverage, 70% fall into high-income earning brackets.[12] And even then it's not a free ride, as many are still expected to contribute to the rising costs of their coverage by paying higher deductibles and/or monthly contributions.

Companies have been aware and scared of these rising health-care costs for years and have lobbied the U.S. government to implement real change in the form of public health policy and benefits. The passing of the Affordable Care Act (Obamacare) in 2010 was the first large-scale public policy, which applied real benefits to ease the strain of employer-paid healthcare and pass on more affordable options to individuals. Open enrollment began in October 2013, and the data available to discern its successful (or unsuccessful) implementation is still years in the making, yet numbers have shown that people who were previously uninsured now have healthcare coverage due to the act.

The collective consciousness agrees on the need for improved public health, and this dawning has been the catalyst for other healthcare initiatives from influential Americans. Some programs, such as Michelle Obama's *Let's Move* initiative to raise a healthier, less obese generation of kids have been well received. However, some have created public vitriol, such as former New York City mayor Michael Bloomberg's proposal to ban sugary drinks larger than 16 ounces.

While both initiatives have sparked conversation and even celebrity endorsements, as in the case of the *Let's Move* initiative (hey Beyoncé), they also touch at the heart of the U.S. healthcare scenario: we are not taking care of ourselves even when more and more is being expected of us in all aspects of our lives. As a 47-hour workweek society, we drink 3.1 cups of coffee a day,[13] 130 million of us are not getting enough sleep,[14] and 26% are still going to work every day even though we feel completely burnt out.[15]

No matter your political affiliation or what you contribute to your traditional healthcare plan, wellness spending, which includes the food, fitness, spa, alternative medicine, and travel industries in addition to workplace wellness, topped a $3.4 trillion global spend in 2013.[16] $3.4 *trillion*! People are clearly looking for something outside of the traditional healthcare model to feel better, function better, and just live better.

Try These Simple Workplace Wellness Tips Right Now

- **Work in 90-minute intervals**—Uninterrupted short work sessions help you to avoid exhaustion. Reward your work with a break allowing for renewal.
- **Take a stroll**—Researchers at the University of Birmingham found that a walk can immediately change your mood for the better and provide improved ability to handle stress at work.
- **Turn off your phone**—Shuck that Pavlovian response and take control of whom you talk to and when. Start doing this simultaneously with your 90-minute work intervals and challenge yourself to extend it.

In case you haven't noticed, your job-related stress triggers don't stop just because you've left the office. No one works 9 to 5 anymore. One of the greatest inventions of the last decade, the smartphone, is also the largest modern-day contributor to our anxiety and hyper alertness. Like a slot machine, we are now conditioned to check our phone every time we see a notification, hear a ding, or feel a vibration—even when what is coming through is junk.

The age of boasting about your ability to multitask is dead. Eating at your desk while answering emails, talking on the phone, and checking Facebook is still happening, but with minimum retention—effectively making your workday twice as long with half the results. Studies now show that multitasking contributes to short-term memory loss, as the cost of switching gears between multiple tasks means you're never fully engaged in one area of concentration.

In a 2012 workplace study, University of California Irvine researchers found that workers who have their email systems set to notify them every time a new email arrives were in a perpetual state of high alert, with correlating higher resting heart rates than those who did not have constant access to their email.[17] This addiction to always being occupied, combined with mounting lifestyle stressors, contributes to the latest workplace loss of productivity defined as presenteeism.

Presenteeism—being physically present at work, but under performing due to illness, stress, and distraction.

American author Mark Twain coined the term "presentee" in his 1892 book *The American Claimant*,[18] and the concept was later popularized in the 2004 *Harvard Business Review* article "Presenteeism: At Work—But Out of It." This broad-spectrum phrase covers a range of issues that have an adverse effect on your time in the office: allergies, chronic disease, stress, financial strain, and family health issues.

While it is difficult to quantify, according to the Integrated Benefits Institute, presenteeism accounts for three times more[19] lost work time than absenteeism—not being at work in the first place. To your employer, this means if workers take an average of 5 sick days a year, an additional 15 days of work are lost to presenteeism. Considering the cost of direct healthcare benefit payouts, it is less expensive to send someone to the doctor to "fix" a problem than to let an undiagnosed indirect health issue linger untreated.

Presenteeism is a new area of study, so questions around how to evaluate causes and create preventative measures are still being formulated. Yet one thing is for sure: if presenteeism is ignored for an extended period of time, it turns into more frequent absenteeism.

So, how should you (and your employer) combat this phenomenon? Strategic renewal. Allow for daytime workouts, better quality of sleep, true nonworking vacation time, and digital detoxes—these are all ways to reduce your overall stress levels and refocus and renew your concentration levels, energy, creativity, and zest for life. While the general consensus is that one's overall well-being is an individual responsibility, companies are now beginning to admit that since you spend most of your waking hours at the office or thinking about work, they need to offer programming, flexible time, and real-world tools to help combat workplace stress in a tangible way.

The Global Wellness Institute estimates that today workplace wellness is a $41 billion industry, with only 25% of large companies offering on-site wellness programming.[20] Many consider a lunch-and-learn education session workplace wellness and go on to provide no additional programming or implementation. This leaves 75% of us having to fend for ourselves until companies catch up with the trend.

Obviously, not all wellness programs are created equal. A survey of current workplace wellness shows today's platforms typically focus on weight loss, smoking cessation, subsidies for gym memberships, and online marketing tools that provide tips for healthier living. Johnson & Johnson, a leading U.S.-based consumer health company, has implemented wellness programming using the above focuses for more than 35 years. Representatives for the company have said that providing wellness programing for over 125,000 employees has saved the company millions of dollars in healthcare costs[21] when it comes to chronic illnesses like obesity, high blood pressure, high cholesterol, and tobacco use.

Currently, the biggest issue workplace wellness faces is that work/life management programs are still being lumped together with illness/disease management programs under the overall healthcare umbrella. While they are in fact all wellness, the statistical data as it relates to healthcare really only offers hard results in terms of quantifiable healthcare claims for illnesses: Did you lose weight? Did you stop smoking? Did you use your gym membership? At present, there is very little hard data available on the corporate integrative programs (yoga, meditation, nutrition consulting, creative writing sessions) which center on prevention and individual lifestyle management/stress reduction programming. Remember, our healthcare system has created habits related to both health and cost which reinforce that the only time you see the doctor is when you are unwell. No hard data can be provided for the times you do not see the doctor because you feel great.

Yet empirical evidence supports the claim that an overall wellness approach toward health creates positive well-being. Case in point: I started to create and prioritize my own wellness routine—yoga, meditation, less meat, less sugar, weekly cardiovascular exercise, and dietary changes instead of over-the-counter medicines, fast foods, and couch sitting. I felt great and got sick less often. After a 3-year absence, I called my own physician to make an appointment. She had put my medical records in storage. She thought I moved.

While there is no formally defined across-the-board definition for workplace wellness programs, the most comprehensive study available to date is the 2013 RAND Workplace Wellness Study, which was sponsored by the U.S. Department of Labor and the U.S. Department of Health and Human Services.

The RAND study is steeped in controversy due to its limited research and sampling, as well as its focus on high-cost health program (i.e., old-school) offerings such as health screenings and blood analysis. These programs are not fun, social, or interactive, but instead are a turn-off to employee participation, so companies have to turn to financial penalties that shame people into participation.

But some interesting statistics arose: 67% of employers cite poor health habits of employees as the top company challenge when it comes to maintaining affordable healthcare.[22] Employees who did participate in the wellness programs had their healthcare costs rise more slowly than those who did not participate. And while only 2% of the participating companies reported actual healthcare savings as a result of the workplace wellness programs, the overall sentiment is that a long-term company and personal investment is worth it.

While there is no factor-to-factor ROI (return on investment) correlation for the lifestyle management programs that take a holistic approach and focus on overall stress reduction in any of today's studies, HR and executive management in companies who use the programs state that the overall gains in positive work culture and employee engagement stemming from workplace wellness programs are worth long-term commitments and may even outweigh any of the hard financial savings. Across the board, employers overwhelmingly agree that *well* employees stay loyal to their companies and have higher morale,[23] which is good for business.

The lack of hard data has not deterred many cutting-edge technology companies whose corporate culture is based around the computer from creating specialized wellness programming within their workspace. In 2007, Google pioneered the way when it created a course for their employees called *Search Inside Yourself*, which takes a science-based approach to developing positive mental habits that contribute to long-lasting well-being. The course, created by Google employee and Jolly Good Fellow (yes, that is his title) Chade-Meng Tan, targets mindfulness and emotional intelligence by providing foundational skills to enhance one's mental clarity, reduce stress, improve creativity, improve communication, and increase overall engagement. The course became so successful that it grew into a spin-off company, which develops and offers 2-day to 4-week programs implemented via lectures, coaching sessions, one-on-one support, and retreat experiences. The well-received curriculum is now taught at companies across the world from Farmers Insurance to Ford Motors.

Wellness works, and top-down leadership who reap its benefits are guaranteed to set a positive example. But if you're dedicated to a company that hasn't quite figured out just how to effectively offer wellness, take charge and be the leader. A culture of wellness is viral. According to Tevis Trower, founder of Balance Integration, one of the first U.S. companies to help large-scale corporations implement workplace wellness programs, worker perception of employer support is key: "What employees wrestle with more than anything is the amount of courage and self-respect it takes to allocate any time to self-care during the day in the throes of surviving in corporate America."[24]

Job-related stress is a big underlying factor in many of our lifestyle illnesses that manifest both inward and outward. Depression and weight gain are areas that have a direct cause and effect on your daily engagement. "You can clearly correlate stress to weight gain," Philip Hagen, an assistant professor of medicine at the Mayo Clinic in Rochester, Minnesota, told *Health Magazine* in a 2012 interview.[25]

A 2013 Harris Interactive study conducted for website Career-Builder showed that 41% of people have gained weight at their current jobs.[26] Long hours of sitting behind a desk with little or no physical activity are an underlying factor, on which we then pile workplace stress. When our body gets stressed, our

Stand Out as a Workplace Wellness Leader and Pitch These Ideas to HR

- **Ban digital devices from meetings**—Get through more material in less time, as you will have everyone's undivided attention.
- **Create renewal zones in the office**—Set up meditation areas, nap zones, or an indoor garden to take people out of their cubical environment and into some new headspace.
- **Restock the kitchen/vending machines with healthy snack choices**—Conditioning people to stop eating as a stress response is going to take time. Aid the consumer of healthier foods by providing fresh fruit, nuts, and protein for high-nutrient fuel-efficient options.

levels of cortisol, an adrenal gland hormone, increase. This rush of energy has been shown to drive people toward eating—particularly foods that are high in sugar and fat.[27] So getting up to stretch or go for a walk breaks up the day and is an investment in your personal wellness, which is beneficial for both you and your employer and allows for higher engagement. When you are more engaged at work, your performance is buoyed, and potential revenue earnings increase 2.5 times over an employee with low engagement.[28]

In 2003, the *Journal of the American Medical Association* released a report showing that employee depression affected U.S. companies to the tune of $34 billion a year in reduced performance at work.[29] If job stress is contributing this much to employees being unwell, companies need to take the first step toward implementing real change.

But the question is—when?

Change on a large scale can be slow, and until employers understand that offering wellness education and implementation is a low-cost expenditure compared to the direct medical costs associated with long-term disease management, the responsibility falls on, guess who: *you.* And who better to experiment with the myriad of wellness offerings out there and pick the components that resonate in a fun and fulfilling way. There is yoga for every personality type, juice shops popping up like Starbucks, meditation rooms in airports, and hotels offering everything from run concierges to specially designed Stay Well® rooms. The world of wellness is becoming versatile, convenient, and sometimes downright wacky, all in the name of bringing out the best version of the only person you'll ever really have: yourself.

MILLENNIALS AND THE FUTURE

> *One of the huge mistakes people make is that they try to force an interest on themselves. You don't choose your passions; your passions choose you.*[30]
>
> —Jeff Bezos, CEO of Amazon.com

Wellness is not a secondary part of life if you are under the age of 35. The generation born between 1980 and 2000 does not view wellness as something you do if there is time. The millennial generation actively invests in healthy living, and America has started to take notice in a big way.

Millennials are trendsetters' and advertisers' most coveted demographic for a reason: they make up 25% of the population and represent $200 billion in annual buying power.[31] American pop culture and big business is already in on the action. Any number of TV spots point to wellness seeping into our societal consciousness, from a commercial for Aflac Insurance set in a yoga class, to Jeff Bridges OM'ing for active rest in a Squarespace spot, to characters on *Law & Order* taking "time off" to attend a yoga retreat in Costa Rica. You cannot escape the wellness phenomenon that has emerged in the last decade.

The education of wellness for this generation has been led by boomers' need to provide a healthier life for the future generations. Millennials are taught from a young age not to diet, but instead to question what you consume in the first place. High schools have been increasingly prohibiting junk food in vending machines, cafeterias, and at after-school programs.[32] All this

Attention Corporate Leaders

U.S. business surveys estimate that presenteeism costs companies upward of $150 billion each year.[1] Reduced production, lost sales, and poor customer services are some of the measurable outcomes that presenteeism has been shown to affect. Working when you're not fully present due to illness or distraction often leads to reduced quantity and poor quality of work. And in some cases, serious mistakes, such as a decimal point in the wrong place, can have repercussions for years to come.

If corporations are serious about investing in wellness—and many are, as a Fidelity Investment & National Business Group health report shows that workplace wellness spending doubled in the past five years[2]—providing engaging programming is just one piece of the puzzle. Both a 2010 Texas A&M University study and the 2013 RAND Workplace Wellness Study reached the same conclusions: in order for real sustained change to take hold in a company, the following six pillars need to be present and continuously maintained:

Strategic Alignment—Healthcare and its associated costs differ from industry to industry and from organization to organization. Therefore, any wellness programming should evaluate the current workplace situation and then be created to fall in line with a company's current and future goals and aspirations, effectively showing participants what they are collectively working toward. Everyone relates to wellness programming on a personal level; therefore, by showing the employee how their wellness contributes to the future of the company, they feel invested in helping to work toward those collective goals.

Communication—A clear internal marketing message needs to be created and adopted across the board, with real resources dedicated to informing and updating employees. Nonverbal communication is also a key—simple workplace steps such as making the stairs more accessible and restocking vending machines with healthy snacks clearly communicates a company's commitment toward improved health.

Opportunity—Programming should be convenient in both location (on-site) and hours (prework, lunch, postwork). The in-your-face approach will show employees that it doesn't take that much additional effort to participate.

Broad Scope in Programming—Currently, most programs focus on measureable data offerings, like weight loss or smoking cessation. This is a great start, but often other ailments such as stress, anxiety, depression, and insomnia are present, as are even more personal life issues such as divorce, deaths in family, or financial well-being, all of which contribute to presenteeism. Corporations need to recognize that there are a wide range of wellness experts and programming available and should consider adding these to the offering.

Engaged Leadership—Watching the company CTO implement walking meetings or hearing the CEO declare that bike racks will be installed in the front of the building shows great leadership and commitment to workplace wellness. Yet there is a very clear disconnect between top-tier management and entry-level employees, as oftentimes middle managers do not provide the support system needed for the programing to be successful. It is up to the company leaders to let employees know they can participate without penalty and actively encourage them to do so.

Continuous Evaluation—Companies change, management changes, people change. Wellness programming is constantly evolving and improving, and the only way to understand whether the programs and the manner in which they are being offered are successful is by soliciting feedback from those who participate.

When these six pillars are successfully implemented, 87% of employees are less likely to leave their companies than their disengaged counterparts.[3] This can account for huge company savings when viewed in the scope of new hires and training.

NOTES

1. Hemp, Paul, "Presenteeism: At Work—But Out of It," *Harvard Business Review*, October 2004.
2. Emerman, Ed, "Companies Are Spending More on Corporate Wellness Programs but Employees Are Leaving Millions on the Table," *Business Group Health*, March 26, 2015.
3. Corporate Leadership Council, "Driving Performance and Retention Through Employee Engagement," 2004, http://www.usc.edu/programs/cwfl/assets/pdf/Employee%20engagement.pdf

early health education has led millennials to have a strong distrust of our current healthcare (illness) system.

Despite this surge in health consciousness, the millennial generation still reports stress at levels that exceed the national average[33] and growing dissatisfaction with both the physical and mental healthcare options available. The 2014 *Communispace* Healthcare Without Borders consumer study showed half of this generation feels that the U.S. government, backed by greedy pharmaceutical lobbies, is to blame for our dysfunctional healthcare system.[34] This insight has pushed millennials outside the traditional healthcare model to seek alternative medicine and wellness as complementary care in an attempt to personalize their well-being and reduce their overall healthcare costs in order to feel like the best version of themselves.

Secure job futures look bleak, as reports surface stating that ready, willing people are available, but there are not enough jobs out there to employ them. With mounting debt, the millennials who are currently employed, even if unhappily, are doing whatever they can to prove their worth and company loyalty: working excess hours, making themselves constantly available on their digital devices, even pulling the weight of two positions just to improve their chances of job security.

As the most overscheduled generation yet, it's no wonder that headlines like "Why Millennial Women Are Burning Out at Work by 30" and others like it have been splashed across the pages of Forbes Magazine, have played out in the national news, and are cause for real concern in the workplace today. This generation visits the doctor less often, self-diagnoses online, turns to home remedies and social media for healthcare solutions, and was the first to adopt wearable healthcare tracking devices.[35] Millennials are more interested in getting a massage, practicing meditation, buying organic food, and using natural nontoxic products than they are taking a quick-fix pill or getting routine healthcare screenings.[36] And they just may have gotten it right.

ARE YOU ALREADY ON THE BRINK OF BURNOUT?

> *If you feel burnout setting in, if you feel demoralized and exhausted, it is best, for the sake of everyone, to withdraw and restore yourself. The point is to have long-term perspective.*[37]
>
> —His Holiness the Dalai Lama

Take a moment for a quick 5-step self-evaluation.

1. **Sleep**—Would you generally say that you are not getting enough sleep or hours of quality rest?
2. **Eating Habits**—Do you lose your appetite when you're busy or reach for the unhealthiest option to cope in what seems like an unmanageable situation?
3. **Exercise**—You know movement is the way to counteract the ill-effects of our increasing sedentary lifestyle. Do you find yourself overwhelmed with the thought of adding exercise to your schedule?
4. **Coping Mechanisms**—Do you lash out at others over minor issues? Do you fire off emails that you later regret?
5. **Success**—Are there never enough hours in your day to complete everything on your list? Do you forget to stop and celebrate the small victories because you bypass them on your way to the next thing?

If you answered yes to more than half of the above questions, congratulations, your fight-or-flight response is in a constant state of readiness for action. You are stressed and making your body and mind work overtime. You may already be on the brink of burnout. Recognizing that you are under stress and that it is affecting all areas of your life is crucial to devising a management strategy.

While companies across the United States are starting to understand the benefits of wellness, acknowledging that there is a problem and implementing a strategy to educate and offer programing with a supportive environment to foster to the work are on different ends of the spectrum. We are living in a world where self-responsibility is the key. As employers cut back on their benefit offerings, individuals are not going to be able to cover their own sickness costs without bankrupting themselves.

Wellness is a personal journey with no one-size-fits all solution. Healthcare costs will continue to rise to unimaginable levels. Preventive care is the only solution that allows you to take responsibility for your own well-being in a way that excites and fulfills you. And while it would be great to have the support and encouragement of your company behind you, the ultimate goal is to change your own behaviors and implement realistic, sustainable self-management techniques in order to improve your quality of life.

Unfortunately, struggling with work-health balance today sends most of us in a beeline for the doctor's office looking for a prescription, a quick fix . . . instead of reexamining our lifestyle. But what else are you supposed to do, right? You spend too much of your life sitting behind a desk, staring at your smartphone, shuttling between business trips, and trying to turn it all off when you get home as it is—how can you expect you to add "well-being" to your stuffed-to-bursting schedule?

Well, here's the kicker: you already have.

Yep. By picking up this book, your road to wellness has already begun. You are now your own agent of change.

While productivity may be hard to quantify as we are producing less and less tangible products in the United States, we can turn to surveys, anecdotal evidence, and significant increases in wellness spending, all of which support consistent claims that if you are left unwell, stressed, distracted, or sick, your positive impact at work and on your own life will suffer.

In order to tackle a true lifestyle change that will allow you to reap the benefits for years to come—think antiaging, longevity of good health, delaying serious age-related diseases—you have to set yourself up for success. It's all about baby steps. The mind is a powerful thing, and by just deciding you want to be on the path to health, happiness, and a longer life, you're already creating momentum. You've just opened up your map and now it's time to take your first steps.

INTERVIEW: Workplace wellness with Tevis Trower, founder of Balance Integration

Growing up with self-professed hippy parents set Tevis Trower on the path toward wellness from a young age. While other kids were sitting in front of the television and eating sugary cereal for breakfast, she learned about exercise, meditation, and the nutritional properties of food. For Tevis, rebelling meant getting an MBA and heading straight for corporate America. After witnessing many workplace implosions, Trower decided to form Balance Integration, one of the first national companies to help large-scale corporations implement workplace wellness programs in order to help combat rising stress levels in employees and attrition for employers.

Working in corporate America gave you a new perspective on what it meant to be an adult and provided you insider experience on what it meant to burn out. What was the most revelatory concept you saw?

Tevis Trower: Year after year all around me people kept dropping like flies. I would watch successful people, people who appeared to have everything from the outside—the job, the salary, the family, the possessions—and they would struggle with the simple question: "Why am I not happy?" It struck me that our culture has set up happiness at work to be a 4-letter word. The overall view is that happiness is fleeting—a moving target—because we should always be focused on what's next.

After this realization, how did the corporate environment change for you?

TT: I started to pay attention to my own well-being and to observe the well-being of those around me. I saw that when people, myself included, were proactively attending to their symptoms—anxiety, restlessness, feeling overwhelmed—issues such as coworker conflicts and absenteeism would resolve themselves. I already had my yoga teaching certification, which is what I was using as a springboard to my own wellness and as a basis to ask myself what frame of mind I needed to move through my day in the happiest, healthiest way possible.

In 2001, I left my corporate job to start Balance Integration and was able to work with the Human Resource teams at AOL, Google, and Yahoo to begin implementing the first workplace wellness programs that dealt with overall lifestyle management. Part of what propelled these large companies' interest in these programs was that they wanted to be the first to introduce this concept. Wellness programming projected an image of cutting-edge cool, and they attracted potential hires and sent a clear message of "You Matter Here"; this soon gave way to instinctively understanding that corporate culture in America was about to shift. These companies acknowledged that stress and burnout and pulling all-nighters were happening, and there were not currently effective tools within the organization to deal with these things.

Workplace wellness has been embraced on many levels and offers all kinds of tailor-made programming. With rising U.S. healthcare costs and recently released statistics showing that 5% of all Google searches are about health and wellness, how are corporations determining their responsibility versus individual responsibility when it comes to wellness?

TT: Unwell employees are costing companies money. When you survey workers in corporate America, they site their top two causes of stress to be money and work. Seventy percent of absenteeism can be tied back to stress-related illnesses.[38] The estimated cost of family health insurance premiums is projected to equal the median household income by 2033.[39] This translates into lost profits, and therefore, the overall trend in corporate America is away from employer paid insurance—it's just an unsustainable cost. The onus is falling more and more on the individual to manage his or her own well-being.

Corporations are realizing that there are loads of information available on how to improve your health and well-being, but when employees are working 10-hour days, there is no time to explore the options. In cutting back on healthcare contributions, companies are stepping forward to give employees access to tools and information that will provide a sense of empowerment. The corporate HR departments and wellness facilitators are striving to offer these programs and implement them from the top level of CEOs down to the junior-most employee so that real cultural change can be implemented and a support system can be created at the office to foster a more well-working environment.

Are corporate wellness programs working?

TT: This is a hard question to answer because there is very limited scientific factor-to-factor correlation, and each corporation approaches its workplace wellness programs differently with different measurable outcomes. What we do know from surveying and having the opportunity to work consistently with large corporations is that programs implemented that support change in the working environment have shown a decrease in rates of attrition and absenteeism as well as a rise in employee engagement.

2

GET REST

I roll over, blink, open my eyes, and wonder where I am. A smile spreads across my face when I realize I'm in my apartment, lying on the couch with sun streaming in through the windows. I reach for my phone to see what time it is.

Crap, it's 4pm. And I just napped for 2 hours. Again.

Sitting up to stretch, I shake the sleep from my head and drink a glass of water while I wonder if I'll be able to fall asleep tonight at a normal time. Turns out I will have no problem curling up in bed at 11pm and sleeping a restful 8 hours.

This was my routine for the first 2 years of my solopreneur life. Every afternoon my mind would start to wander, I'd begin to fall asleep at my desk, and instead of reaching for a cup of coffee, I'd head to the couch to take a nap. Call me lazy. Call me sleep-deprived. Either way, working from home allowed me to set my own schedule, enabling me to pay back the sleep debt I accumulated from years of running myself ragged. Now, 4 years later, I no longer nap, I sleep between 7 and 8 restful hours every night, and most mornings I wake up just before my alarm sounds.

I didn't know it at the time, but years of sacrificing sleep in order to work more hours and to say yes to more social events was not only making me cranky and contributing to my ill-health; it was also increasing my stress level and leaving me unfocused. It turns out that even with a 2-hour break in the middle of the day, I was completing more productive hours of work than ever, as I felt more focused and more rested than I'd been in years.

COUNTING SHEEP

The worst thing in the world is to try to sleep and not to.

—Unknown

If you've ever laid in bed counting sheep or trying to perfect a full body relaxation exercise and gotten nowhere, you know you're in for a long night. Sleep helps the brain remove toxic proteins from its neurons, restoring the ability to process information and problem solve as well as regulate stress and emotional reactivity.[1]

Our bodies crave sleep, and the brain starts to fog or shut down when we don't get enough of it. Yet there are plenty of outside influences that not only keep us awake, but that we use to trick our bodies into putting off rest. Computer screens, lack of physical exertion throughout the day, experiencing pain from a chronic health issue, side effects from medication, and feeling depressed or anxious are all real things that can interfere with sleep. "Worrying prompts your body to produce the adrenaline-like chemical epinephrine, which keeps you awake," says Joyce Walsleben, associate professor of medicine at the New York University School of Medicine.[2] When you are in a state of arousal from anxiety, it constricts the blood vessels, making your extremities cold. Cold hands and cold feet contribute to keeping the body on high alert, as it's easier to fall asleep when your whole body is warm.

Coffee is an obvious culprit that helps to wake us up and keep us awake, since caffeine increases adrenaline production and keeps the brain in a semi-awake state. With caffeine having a 6-hour half-life,[3] it's no wonder the added soda, energy drinks, or decaf coffee (which still has about 3% caffeine in it) consumed throughout the day is one of the reasons you're staring at the ceiling when you head to bed.

Are You Affected by a Sleep Disorder?

It is estimated that 1/3 of U.S. adults experience some kind of sleep difficulties throughout the week.[1] Could trouble in these sleep areas be stealing your precious hours of shut-eye and productivity?

- **Sleep Inertia**—The period between waking up and feeling fully awake. It can take anywhere from 2 to 4 hours for sleep inertia to fade completely.
- **Sleep Latency**—Time spent in bed awake between when you turn out the lights and when you actually fall asleep.
- **Sleep Apnea**—Collapsing of the body's airways, which causes short pauses in breathing. This can happen many times throughout the night without you knowing it, but it manifests in feeling sleepy throughout the day.
- **Insomnia**—Encompasses a host of sleep issues: prolonged sleep latency, sleep apnea, and inability to return to sleep once awoken. What qualifies a person as having insomnia is when these issues are persistent and occur at least three times a week over a prolonged period of time.

NOTE

1. Roth, T., "Prevalence, Associated Risks, and Treatment Patterns of Insomnia," *Journal of Clinical Psychiatry* 66, Suppl 9 (2005): 10-13, quiz 423.

And what about that glass of wine you poured after a hard day to help you relax? Unfortunately, it may be keeping you up at night too. Alcohol can help facilitate brain shut down and muscle relaxation, but it also works to relax the muscles around the body's airways, which interferes with breathing. This can lead to snoring and even sleep apnea, as the body needs to constantly wake up and change positions to recapture the breath. "Alcohol changes your sleep patterns, and once it clears your system—usually four to five hours after you fall asleep—the brain becomes hyperaroused and you wake up," says Meir Kryger, director of research at the Gaylord Sleep Center at Gaylord Hospital in Wallingford, Connecticut.[4]

NURTURE YOUR NATURE

A day well spent procures a happy sleep.[5]

—Leonardo da Vinci

The root of sleep pattern research began in France in the 1700s when astronomer Jean-Jacques d'Ortous de Mairan observed that the leaves of his heliotrope plant opened and closed at the same time every day. Struck by this fascinating observation, he moved the plant into a space that received no light and found that the plant continued its daily routine even without the influence of the sun.

When the sun rises in the morning, it emits strong short wavelengths of blue light. Our exposure to this light is a natural signal to the body that it is time to be awake and alert. Throughout the day, the sun's rays morph into an amber color before setting and leaving us in semi-darkness. Within this daily cycle, we too adapt, with some of us gravitating more toward mornings while others are night owls. Certain people have more energy during the long days of summer, while less light during the winter months makes some people fatigued and unproductive. Each of us has an underlying biology that predisposes us to a natural circadian rhythm, which becomes our optimal sleep cycle.

Circadian rhythm—a biological process of cyclical changes including body temperature and hormone levels that occur over a 24-hour period and drive our internal clock toward sleep or wake times.

Circadian rhythm research began in the late 1960s with the observation of fruit flies. Scientists noticed that fruit fly eggs always hatched at the same time of day. This discovery led to identifying an internal "clock" gene that is synchronized to environmental stimuli such as light that regulates the activity of the

The Sleep Cycle

One complete sleep cycle runs between 90 and 120 minutes. In a complete phase, you will experience the following stages of sleep:

- **Drowsiness**—During this stage, your body begins to transition from being fully awake to shutting down parts of your body and mind, so you can begin to fall asleep.
- **Light Sleep**—Eye movement begins to cease, muscles relax, and your consciousness ebbs as you fully drift off.
- **Non-REM Sleep** Here, your body's physiological activity slows down. Brain waves get slower, breathing and heart rate are reduced, and blood pressure drops. If you've ever woken up during this stage, you'll remember feeling groggy and disoriented.
- **REM Sleep**—This is our deepest level of sleep with intense brain activity. Our eye movements become more rapid, our heart rate increases, and we enter into a dream state. This is the stage of sleep that allows our body to recover most.

gene.[6] Since each of us has a unique DNA structure, our genes actually dictate how much sleep we need.[7]

Before the advent of electricity, people relied upon the rising and setting of the sun to define nondrowsy waking hours. Neuroscience professor Dr. Joseph Takahashi says there is a genetic component that coordinates with the earth's biology and helps to regulate the sleep and wake cycles in each of us. This component, the suprachiasmatic nucleus, a group of regulatory cells located in the hypothalamus section of the brain, operates on a 24-hour cycle and controls our sleep functions, making us feel sleepy or awake.[8] As our ancestors got busier and societal needs developed beyond the waking hours that the sun could provide, fires, candles, and gas lanterns aided in extending the hours during which we had the ability to see. Eventually, light bulbs were invented. All of these light extenders, which emit long-wavelength infrared light or incandescent light, allowed our active hours to lengthen and our sleeping hours to shrink, shifting our biological sleep patterns.

The body's regular sleep cycle alternates between light and deep sleep. During sleep, the brain quiets down, the heart rate slows, and blood pressure falls, all things that help the body to relax. One to two hours before bedtime, our bodies begin to release a hormone called melatonin. The release of melatonin, made by the pineal gland in the brain, correlates with the light and dark cycle of the earth, which tells our bodies when it's time to sleep and when it's time to wake. Normally, we go through 4 to 6 sleep cycles each night before melatonin production slows and the body starts to reboot, increasing its core temperature and sending cortisol (a steroid hormone) into the system, readying it for morning about an hour before we wake up.

Exposing the body to light during the hours when it's dark outside interrupts the natural production of melatonin and sends signals to the body to stay awake. This is how we are able to shift our circadian rhythm (sometimes painfully) when traveling across time zones. People who work the night shift also use this method to train their bodies to stay awake forgoing the cycles of the earth that are telling them to sleep. Till Roenneberg, a professor of chronobiology at Ludwig-Maximilians University in Munich, discovered that training your body to stay awake for the night shift stresses your internal systems, specifically the immune system, which is one of the reasons that night-shift workers suffer a higher than normal rate of cancer, diabetes, heart conditions, and other chronic diseases.[9]

Today, it is common to regulate sleep cycles to fit into a 9am to 6pm workday, as life happens around us when the sun is out. As the body picks up the environmental cues of light and sound, the internal biological clock starts to adjust its release of hormones. Soon body temperature, blood pressure, and melatonin release are regulated into a 24-hour cycle. While our internal clock isn't perfectly correlated with the external surroundings, it is believed that as humans we learned evolutionary adaptation: syncing our bodily cycles to the environmental cycles that happen around us.[10]

In the 1980s, historian A. Roger Ekirch began researching sleep cycles after he uncovered multiple journals, diaries, and medical books, along with classic literature pieces going back to Homer's *Odyssey*, that referenced something called "first sleep"

Check Your Meds

Medication, both prescription and over-the-counter, can come with a long list of side effects. Insomnia or restless sleep is a common reaction to the limited list below. If you are taking any of these medications and have noticed your sleep pattern change, please consult your doctor.

ADHD Medication: Adderall, Dexedrine, Ritalin
Anti-Smoking Medication: Chantix, Nicorette, Wellbutrin
Cold and Allergy Medication: Benadryl, Claritin, NyQuil, Zyrtec
Depression Medication: Lexapro, Paxil, Prozac, Zoloft
Heart and Blood Medication: Betapace, Capoten, Lipitor, Lopressor
Herbal Medication: Ginseng, green tea, St. John's wort
Pain Relief Medication: Excedrin, Sudafed

and "second sleep." In his 2001 book *Sleep We Have Lost*, Ekirch delves into something called segmented sleep: the historical recordings of sleep that happened in two large chunks from 9pm to 12am and again from 3am to 6am. To further his findings, Ekirch consulted psychiatrist Thomas Wehr, who in 1999 published a study in the journal *Neurobiology of Sleep and Circadian Rhythms* showcasing the results of his segmented sleep experiment. Dr. Wehr found that when sequestering his subjects at night and removing artificial light—no TV, no computers, no light bulbs—they naturally reverted into two segmented sleep patterns after just four weeks.[11]

Oftentimes, we ignore or push past the bodily signs that are begging us to shut down and sleep. If you've ever experienced a second wind—that burst of energy that helps you stay awake—you've just tricked your internal clock into skipping, like a record, the prime period for natural sleep to begin. This change can have you reaching for a pill to induce sleep once you're actually ready to lie down, or have you constantly fighting the snooze button in the morning in an effort to try and regain those missed hours and in hopes of re-regulating back to a natural sleep cycle. Both of these temporary solutions will actually make life worse in the long term. Forcing the body to start the sleep cycle or coercing it to wake mid-cycle makes the entire process more difficult to sustain and can leave you waking up feeling worse and less rested than when you started.[12]

Staying out late to socialize or having to wake up early to catch a plane throws our system out of whack. If it's once or twice, the body can recover, but frequently adjusting your sleep pattern can cause a short circuit. Our body doesn't know the difference between a weekday and a weekend; it cannot quickly adjust for an important morning meeting or understand the need to head to bed early in a pinch to feel well-rested if you have a big day tomorrow. Instead, by sticking to a consistent schedule—awake and active when the sun is out and sleepy and sedentary when it's not—the body can establish a healthy circadian rhythm.

BLUE LIGHT SPECIAL

Some of the biggest offenders of sleep deprivation in the modern age are our gadgets, and not just those of a hand-held variety. Today, we sleep less because our brains are too engaged. Add stress, stimulants, and screens to the mix along with our constant exposure to light, and it messes with our natural ability to rest well. Remember the *Seinfeld* episode in which Kramer begs Jerry to switch apartments because the neon chicken sign is constantly shining into his bedroom and disrupting this sleeping? Substitute your smartphone into this scenario and you have the modern day equivalent.

Smart technology is the basis for our modern world playing such an important and often addictive role in our lives; it is no wonder that 68% of owners bring their screens, which emit blue light, to bed with them.[13] A whopping 90% of Americans, myself included, admit to using their blue light-emitting electronics at least 1 hour before bedtime.[14]

Yet it is only in the last 20 years that science has acquired a basic biological understanding of how the eye's retina processes short-wave blue light due to the newly discovered photo pigment melanopsin in the retina.[15] Melanopsin is found in the photoreceptor cells of our eyes and communicates information directly to our brain. If the melanopsin detects blue light, it signals our brain to stop melatonin production and stay awake.

In 2001, *Chronobiology International* published the first study that confirmed the short-wave blue light effect on melatonin production.[16] Once scientists established fact to this working theory, the discussion turned to look at what bodily effects the constant exposure to blue light has on our physical health as well as our sleep patterns.

Anne-Marie Chang, associate neuroscientist in Brigham and Women's Hospital's Division of Sleep and Circadian Disorders, has spent years studying this field. Chang surmised that using a blue light–emitting screen in the early part of the evening, even at low intensity, would suppress the release of melatonin and negatively affect sleep. Her research team gathered test subjects into the sleep laboratory for observation and was able to confirm that those who used tablets before bed took longer to fall asleep and spent less time in their restorative REM stage.[17]

The team then took blood tests from the tablet users to determine whether any biological effects occurred. The results showed that not only did blue light indeed shift the release of melatonin moving the sleep cycle back by 90 minutes, but it also disrupted morning alertness and impaired work performance, health, and overall safety.[18] This pattern of use shows that by using a blue light–emitting device, you are shifting your circadian timing and decreasing your sleepiness in the evening, inevitably pushing back your melatonin production and the feeling of getting sleepy at night.

Worldwide concern over the effect of our digital devices is so great that in 2015, for the first time, a conference titled "Blue Light Symposium" was held in New York City. Speakers and scientists from Japan, Spain, France, and the United States gathered to discuss light pollution and the adverse effects of blue light exposure. Ophthalmology professor Kazuo Tsubota of Keio University School of Medicine spoke, citing recent studies linking adverse effects of blue light on melatonin levels, which can lead to the development of diabetes and cancer.[19]

Some current ideas that scientists and tech innovators alike are proposing to combat blue light effects are holding devices further away from your face, turning tablets and phones into black/white or night mode, or enabling the Night Shift feature on Apple devices in hopes of allowing regular melatonin production. If you want to go even further, you could use amber-tinted lenses, worn like sunglasses at night, which are believed to block blue light from both screens and energy-efficient light bulbs. All of these potential solutions require further testing in order to confirm their effectiveness, but we will continue to see new technological developments aimed at working around this problem.

With the American Medical Association issuing a policy[20] which recognizes that exposure to excessive blue light exacerbates sleep disorders, and the International Agency for Research on Cancer calling blue light a possible carcinogenic pollution,[21] further studies will be conducted and additional solutions need to be proposed that take our long-term health into consideration. As science continues to catch up with empirical evidence that light pollution changes our sleep/wake patterns, in the coming years we'll see the results of additional blue light studies, which are currently underway and hopefully develop some coping mechanisms that are safe and effective.

YOUR BED IS CALLING

While blue light is absolutely a contributing factor to health and sleep issues, it is rarely the sole cause for sleep disorders. Outside influences such as stress, anxiety, ill-health, or depression can lead you to pick up a screen to cope. In fact, Netflix is counting on your binge-watching (but really, we had to know how *Bloodline* ended!), which can create or contribute to insomnia, making falling asleep tough and staying asleep even more of a challenge.

A 2013 Gallup poll showed that 43% of Americans acknowledged that they would feel better if they got more sleep.[22] And while working adults under the age of 65 report less insomniac episodes, it's been recounted that 30% of U.S. adults have occasional or short-term insomnia.[23] Insomnia can last for days or

Is It Time to Move?

Is where you live causing you to lose sleep? On the basis of the data gathered by the *Centers For Disease Control and Prevention*,[1] these five U.S. states report the highest percentage of adults staring at the ceiling on a nightly basis for the past month due to a variety of issues such as overall stress, the inability to work, a child at home, and obesity issues.

Florida	28.9%
New York	28.5%
Texas	26.6%
Illinois	27.1%
California	24.9%

NOTE

1. Centers for Disease Control and Prevention, "Behavioral Risk Factor Surveillance Survey 2008-2009." www.cdc.gov/BRFSS

stretch on for years, leading to or exacerbate other physical and mental health problems.

It is widely recommended that adults, no matter where in the world they live, get around eight hours of sleep a night in order to stay healthy and perform at optimal levels. The reality is that the average working adult gets about six hours.[24] Oftentimes, the excess coffee and the sugary foods consumed throughout the day to help keep us awake compound our lack of rest. In turn, all that caffeine and sugar leads to difficulty falling asleep at night, creating a habitual cycle that becomes incredibly hard to break.

Dr. Charles Czeisler, a preeminent sleep expert and chief of the Division of Sleep and Circadian Disorders at Brigham and Women's Hospital, has been studying sleep for the last five decades. Throughout his years of research, he has found that the average sleep duration on work nights for adults has decreased by 90 minutes since the 1950s.[25] On average, this deprives our bodies of one full sleep cycle a night compared to our parent's generation.

International Incidents Caused by Lack of Sleep

Think missing a few nights of good sleep is not that big a deal? Unfortunately, some of the most horrific and deadly accidents in history have occurred due to lack of sleep.

- **Exxon Valdez Oil Spill**—In 1989, one of the most devastating man-made environmental disasters resulted in over 11 million gallons of crude oil spilled into the Gulf of Alaska. The commission that investigated the accident found that workers on the ship were sleep-deprived, working up to 18 hours a day preceding the accident.
- **Chernobyl**—To date, over 1 million people have died from cancer-related illnesses traced back to the 1986 nuclear explosion that leaked radioactive poisons into the air. The accident happened in the middle of the night after a worker's 13 hours on the job.
- **Challenger Explosion**—In January 1986, many of us watched in horror as the Challenger space shuttle blew up on live TV. A Presidential Commission charged with investigating the accident discovered human error and poor judgment calls related to early morning shift hours and lack of sleep were responsible.

Why is sleep so important anyway? It improves our mood, our immune system, our eating habits, plus our brains benefit, as sleep is critical for learning. "We integrate the knowledge we gained today with our prior experiences and we rehearse places we've been during the night. We get insight as well." Dr. Czeisler said in his TED Talk.[26] Basically, if we get a good night's sleep, the task(s) we learned today will be better performed tomorrow.

If we consistently get short sleep, our attention, dexterity, and vigilance to details begin to suffer. If we cheat ourselves out of a full night of rest more than two nights in a row, then larger issues such as obesity and even premature death can start to develop.[27] But what if you short yourself sleep Monday–Friday and then sleep in late to make up for it during the weekend? According to a study published in the *Journal of Sleep Research*, the brain's restricted operational capacity will still affect your performance for several days following the weekend "recovery."[28]

Any new parent can understand what it's like to be sleep-deprived. Stumbling around, unable to concentrate, your judgment is impeded. Forget solving any major problems. To an outsider who doesn't know you have a new baby at home, you may appear drunk. Well, it turns out if you are regularly getting 4 to 5 hours of sleep a night, your level of cognitive impairment is on par with someone who *is* legally drunk.[29]

Did you commute to work today? Do you remember your journey, every part in detail? No? We've all had moments like this, not remembering how you got somewhere but arriving safely, or going back into the house or another room to grab something you forgot but getting there and having no clue what you were supposed to be looking for. The National Heart, Lung and Blood Institute developed a name for this: microsleep, which refers to brief moments of sleep that occur when you're normally awake.[30] You can't control microsleep and you might not even be aware it is happening. Clifford Saper, head of Neurology at Beth Israel Deaconess Medical Center, equates these incidents to an intermittent power failure of the brain.[31] On the surface, this might not seem like a huge deal, but in the United States drowsy drivers are responsible for a 1/5 of all car accidents and around 8,000 deaths a year.[32] With an estimated 80,000 drivers falling asleep at the wheel every day, these are numbers we cannot afford to ignore.

"I'll sleep when I'm dead,"[33] quipped singer-songwriter Warren Zevon in his 1976 rock hit, a sentiment which has been adopted for generations by ambitious workaholics the world over. While this cheeky statement is used to justify continuous waking hours, what Zevon probably did not understand is that death may find you sooner if you cut your sleep time.

Our body's immune system relies on sleep to stay healthy so that it can fight harmful bacteria and common infections. In the 1980s, sleep researchers at the University of Chicago kept rats awake 24/7 in order to study the effects of insomnia and sleep deprivation. The rats started to show signs of impending death eleven days into the experiment and at four weeks started to die.[34] "The longer you sleep, the better off you are, the less susceptible you are to colds," Sheldon Cohen, who studies the effects of stress on health at Pittsburgh's Carnegie Mellon University, said after completing a study which showed that people who sleep fewer than 7 hours a night are three times more likely to contract a cold than those who average 8 hours.[35] And colds are just the tip of the iceberg when it comes to health problems associated with lack of sleep. Inadequate sleep has been linked to chronic diseases including diabetes, cardiovascular disease, obesity, and depression.

Sleep, an active physiological process, actually helps your body to conserve energy and resources, allowing it to focus on areas that need to be repaired and restored. When we deprive ourselves of a restful night's sleep, heart disease and high blood pressure can develop, skin's collagen begins to break down leaving us looking older,[36] and for men, testosterone levels drop to those associated with someone of older age.[37] Further studies have concluded that people who are continually sleep deprived are at an increased risk of developing dementia.[38]

You may have also noticed that sleep and food are intertwined. The more hours of the day you are awake, the more fuel you tend to consume to keep you going. Shortening the sleep cycle upsets our body's hormone balance as sleep regulates the hormones that control appetite, metabolism, and glucose processing.[39] When hormones are no longer in a healthy balance, we feel hungry and unsatisfied, even if we just ate. Research has found that this continued pattern leads to an increased risk of developing type 2 diabetes; so optimizing sleep duration may be a good way to improve blood sugar.[40]

Too little sleep also means a greater possibility to overeat energy-rich foods that trick our bodies into becoming hungry at odd times creating irregular snacking patterns. "We then eat foods full of sugar, fat, and carbohydrates to give us quick boosts of energy—and then have a harder time stopping. Getting enough sleep—around 7 to 8 hours—stops that negative cycle before it starts,"[41] writes clinical psychologist Shelby Freedman Harris.

If you keep up a steady diet of inflammatory foods (see chapter 6 for a deep dive into these foods and their effects), they could cause acid reflux or lead to more vivid dreams,[42] which disrupts your sleep pattern completely. Developing inflammatory eating habits inevitably leads to weight gain, which can lead to snoring as your lungs or air passageways can become constricted from the added pounds. People who are obese have shorter sleep cycles,[43] which set up cravings for energy-rich food. Poor eating habits that develop during what are supposed to be your regular sleep hours start to have an effect on your brain and memory problems can occur.[44]

After two consecutive nights of short disruptive sleep, I get cranky, emotionally reactive, and easily hungry. Anyone else? It's at that point I revert to answering anything that feels like a big daunting question with a "let me sleep on it" response, ultimately putting off or avoiding making a decision in the first place. Turns out I'm not alone and there is actually a name for this: decision fatigue. Without realizing it, I instinctively knew that sleep would make my decision-making powers stronger and clearer.

Decision fatigue, a term coined by social psychologist Roy F. Baumeister,[45] happens as the body and brain grow tired throughout the day. The more decisions we make, the more taxing it becomes on the brain. Eventually, we feel overloaded and start looking for ways to make faster choices. When you are sleep deprived or stressed, these decisions can become impulsive or reckless, as you do not expend the appropriate amount of energy to think through all the consequences. (Ask anyone in the public eye who's sent a dick pic). "Even the wisest people won't make good choices when they're not rested and their glucose is low," Baumeister told the New York Times.[46]

Maybe for you sleep deprivation makes you giddy and hyperactive or prone to mood swings. "It's almost as though, without sleep, the brain revert(s) back to more primitive patterns of activity, in that it was unable to put emotional experiences into context and produce controlled, appropriate responses," said Matthew Walker, director of UC Berkeley's Sleep and Neuroimaging Lab.[47]

Walker came to this conclusion after using functional magnetic resonance imaging (fMRI) to study the amygdala, the emotional processing center of the brain. The UC Berkeley study

What Keeps You Up at Night?

A myriad of issues could be keeping you up at night or preventing you from falling asleep in the first place. That lengthy list includes:

Short-Term Sleep Culprits:

- Anxiety, boredom, diet, lack of exercise, medication side effects, stress

Longer-Term Issues:

- Blue light effects, chronic pain, depression, kidney disease, menopause, neurological disorders, nicotine, post-traumatic stress disorder (PTSD), thyroid disease

On the other end of the spectrum, one could oversleep to deal with any of the above issues. While occasionally oversleeping isn't bad, if you are always doing it or have continuous trouble getting out of bed, take note. Sleep issues could be a combination of any of the above, and the symptoms could manifest in different ways. It's best not to jump to conclusions or create a self-diagnosis. Instead make an appointment with a sleep specialist to discuss your current lifestyle and create a plan to begin making changes.

found that participants who stayed awake for 35 straight hours were 60% more emotionally reactive[48] than those who got a full night's sleep. This is because the amygdala goes into overdrive when you function without sleep, which affects the prefrontal cortex of the brain, throwing logical reasoning out the window, and prevents the body from departing the hyperaware fight-or-flight stage. A separate study conducted at the University of Pennsylvania[49] found that when sleep is restricted to 4.5 hours per night for one week, we become mentally exhausted, causing us to feel sad and angry as well as more stressed.

Sleep studies and brain imaging has linked chronic insomnia to lower gray matter density in areas that regulate the brain's ability to make decisions.[50] If sleep cycles or duration improves, not only are decision-making powers enhanced, but also one's ability to problem solve, control emotions, and regulate behavior, as well as resolve countless mental and physical health problems. All of this means getting consecutive good night's sleep will make you happier and healthier.

SLEEP YOUR WAY TO THE TOP

It is a common experience that a problem difficult at night is resolved in the morning after the committee of sleep has worked on it.[51]

—John Steinbeck

My experiences working in the corporate world taught me that many in the chain of command think sleep (like vacation) is a waste of time—something people lacking ambition or the drive to get ahead do. Often the corporate executives or bosses I encountered lived by the "work hard/play hard" mantra putting sleep in the luxury, not necessity, column. This approach made it clear that when they prioritized work over sleep, they became grumpy and even abusive, creating a hostile work environment.

When one is short on sleep, becoming cranky and unfocused or having decision fatigue set in is not an uncommon side effect. In any short sleep situation, you can easily become short-tempered, snapping at someone or have someone snap at you because you're not thinking clearly. Your bad night's sleep is not only negatively affecting you, the person who is sleep-deprived, but it's also affecting the person who bore the brunt of that lack of sleep. Take this scenario into and office setting and amplify it, and you can start to understand how it impacts productivity.

Dr. Ana C. Krieger, a New York City sleep specialist who I interviewed for this book, told me, "It is important to note that a very small percentage of the population can get by with less than 6 hours of sleep."[52] And while successful business leaders

Positive Productivity Starts with the Boss

Want to increase employee productivity throughout the workday preventing presenteeism? Here are the seven ways to institute cultural changes from the top down:

1. **Allow for more frequent breaks**—3 minutes to stand and stretch will refocus the body and mind.
2. **Increase access to natural light**—This will affect people's happiness factor as well as help sync their circadian rhythm.
3. **Provide checklists for rote tasks**—Easy tasks give the brain a break, and if a checklist is handy, then it will not tax memory; therefore, doing the task actually clears the mind.
4. **Encourage strategic renewal**—Daytime workouts, naps, increased vacation time, anything that boots performance during the day leaving night for sleeping.
5. **Offer flexible start times and/or work from home options**—Greater control over personal schedules relieves stress and allows for some extra minutes of shuteye.
6. **Comp weekend workdays**—Working outside normal workdays or adding extra hours can put strain on sleep and increase stress. Give back that time when possible.
7. **Block office emails after 9pm**—Someone sending a late night email shouldn't obligate you to answer it, but often it does. Instead create a boundary and halt email delivery for daylight hours.

such as Twitter founder Jack Dorsey, Yahoo CEO Marissa Mayer, and even former president Bill Clinton have all been reported to get by on less than 6 hours of sleep a night,[53] it's important to not measure yourself against these standards. David Dinges, a psychology professor, reminds us that oftentimes highly successful people can function adequately on less sleep and are "more productive because they don't have to worry about everyday issues like paying for education or saving for retirement and typically have teams of people taking care of mundane life tasks such as laundry, paying bills, and shuttling children to and from activities, which frees them up to have a more singular focus on work."[54]

A study released by the *Centers for Disease Control and Prevention* in 2010 showed that 1/3 of the U.S. workforce, over 40 million people, get less than six hours of sleep each night.[55] Finding this information astounding, Ronald Kessler, sociologist and professor at Harvard Medical School, authored a 2011 study on the financial impact of sleep deprivation and the effects it has on industry. He and his colleagues found that annualized individual-level presenteeism associated with lack of sleep worked out to 11.3 days of lost work performance, and when expanded to include the total U.S. workforce, annual presenteeism resulted in a total of $63.2 billion financial loss.[56]

Financial losses due to sleep deprivation make themselves known in a couple of ways. According to Christopher Barnes, when you are sleep-deprived, it tampers with your self-control and ethics. If a worker gets consecutive short sleep and arrives on the job to fulfill their responsibilities, they are more likely to engage in bad behavior in ways that affect the company's bottom line, such as falsifying expenses or misreporting financial numbers.[57]

What's worse than financial loss... how about death? The last place you want anyone to be sleep-deprived at work would be a hospital, yet doctors who participate in long hours of shift work often fall into this category. Until 2011, it was standard practice to have first-year residents work 30-hour shifts. In 2004, a study led by researchers at Brigham and Women's Hospital found that residents who took on those 30-hour shifts made 36% more serious medical errors than those who worked shifts half as long.[58] There is now a ban on these 30-hour shifts, and in its place there is a 16-hour limit on consecutive work hours.

While working in an office setting isn't necessarily a life or death situation, with companies asking employees to work longer hours, they are also essentially asking employees to sleep less. Fortune 500 companies Goldman Sachs, Johnson & Johnson, and Google are taking sleep deprivation and its effect on productivity seriously. These companies offer health coaching surrounding sleep issues, bringing in sleep experts to consult, and

The Case for Sleeping on the Job

In 2007, Dimitrios Trichopoulos of the Harvard School of Public Health in Boston published the results of a study in the *Archives of Internal Medicine* that touted the health benefits of napping. The study found that those who systematically napped had a 37% lower coronary mortality rate than those who did not.[1]

Arianna Huffington, founder of *The Huffington Post*, wrote in her most recent book *Thrive* about how she collapsed from exhaustion. This experience and subsequent research led to her to champion the benefits of sleep and create nap rooms at the office. She regularly lectures on how sleep deprivation costs businesses too much money and recently launched Thrive Global, a new workplace wellness company that aims to establish practices which will change the way we work today.

In the mid-1990s, NASA conducted a study on napping and found those who napped on the job gained a 16% median increase in reaction time.[2] The U.S. Naval Medical Research center looked at the consequences of sleep loss in pilots and determined that strategic naps were an effective countermeasure for sleep deprivation.[3]

Companies like Nike, Zappos, and Uber have agreed that boosting productivity with a nap instead of an extra cup of coffee is the way to go and have installed naps rooms at their headquarters. If you do not have access to a nap room but are lucky enough to have your own office or access to a quiet space, take 15 minutes each afternoon and use it to refresh. Dim the lights, turn off all your devices, and set an alarm. It might take some training to learn to fall asleep, but once you get into a pattern you'll notice alertness will be restored, your motor skills will be improved, and your mood will be enhanced.[4]

NOTES

1. Trichopoulos, Dimitrios, "Siesta in Healthy Adults and Coronary Mortality in the General Population," *Archives of Internal Medicine* 167, 3 (2007): 296–301. DOI:10.1001/Archinte.167.3.296

2. Rosekind, M. R., "Alertness Management: Strategic Naps in Operational Settings," *Journal of Sleep Research* 4, S2 (December 1995): 62-66. http://www.ncbi.nlm.nih.gov/pubmed/10607214

3. Hartzler, Beth, "Fatigue on the Flight Deck: The Consequences of Sleep Loss and the Benefits of Napping," *Accident Analysis and Prevention* 62 (January 2014): 309-18. DOI: 10.1016/J.Aap.2013.10.010. Epub October 19, 2013

4. Mednick, Sara C., "Comparing the Benefits of Caffeine, Naps and Placebo on Verbal, Motor and Perceptual Memory," *Behavioural Brain Research* 193, 1 (November 3, 2008): 79-86.

have even instituted office hours requiring people to leave for a forced break.[59]

Overall, we're not listening to what bodies are trying to tell us. We push aside the very things that make us function optimally (exercise, healthy food, sleep) in favor of work. Instead of worrying about managing our time into a prescribed set of office hours, maybe it would benefit us to manage our energy and assess when we offer the most productivity.

Aside from work itself, commuting is an activity that competes with sleep. A study published in the *Journal of Sleep*[60] established that those who are self-employed, allowing them to plan their own schedules, had significantly lower odds of being a short sleeper. Additionally, Penn State research found that if you are not self-employed but are given more control over your work hours including flexible schedules, adjustable start times or given the opportunity to work from home some days, you will feel more in control and less stressed, which will increase your nightly sleep time and therefore productivity.[61]

Offering flexible hours or options to work remotely may be a way to solve productivity and sleep deprivation issues, but for many companies, these modifications are just not possible to institute. Offices do have rules against drinking on the job, using drugs, on-site sexual harassment, and a host of other regulations for employee safety. Now that we understand how detrimental lack of sleep can be both to the body and to the bottom line, it's important to create office policies limiting the workday. Monitoring smartphones and responding to colleagues when you should be sleeping ultimately makes everyone less effective, as it sets off the domino effect for an unending workday.[62]

SAY GOODNIGHT, GRACIE

A lot of people engage in sleep procrastination, which is to say they put sleep off, thinking they simply have too much to do to sleep.[63]

—Dr. Michael Breus, The Sleep Doctor

Willing yourself to sleep does not work. Trying to forcefully quiet your brain can actually have the opposite effect and keep you up longer as you lie in bed thinking about all you have to do as well as all the sleep you are missing. The best way to set yourself up for a good night's sleep is to focus on your sleep hygiene: creating good sleep habits.

Sleep hygiene—habits and practices that are conductive to sleeping well on a regular basis.

Your sleep, just like your optimal wellness, is different from one person to the next and can be influenced by everything from lifestyle to socioeconomic status to genes. While there is no magic solution, there are ways to calm your body and prepare it for rest. Giving up or reducing your intake of nicotine, caffeine, and alcohol will decrease stimuli in your body, while sticking to a regular fitness routine will tire the body and relieve stress. Establishing consistent mealtimes as well as waking up at the same time every day will contribute to acclimating your circadian rhythm. Monitoring your exposure to light and shutting down your connection to work a few hours before bed will help to reduce stress. All of these decisions should be made consciously in order to signal to your body that it's time to relax.

There are other mind-body options that can be explored as well. Muscle and music relaxation techniques have shown to improve sleep efficiency,[64] yoga can be used to decrease insomnia,[65] and even regularly playing the didgeridoo, an Australian wind instrument, has been shown to be an effective treatment for

Ten Get-Ready-for-Sleep Tips

Try adding these tips to your day and see if they may work as part of your new sleep routine:

- Eat a light dinner
- Shut off the TV and computer 1 hour before bed
- Make a calendar appointment to sleep and keep it
- Leave your phone in the living room
- Take a bath before bed
- Journal before bed
- Reserve your bed for sleep and sex—no other activities
- Invest in a foam mattress so you don't feel your partner move
- Do a 10 minute yoga for sleep sequence
- Play soothing music or mantras

people who deal with sleep apnea, as it stiffens the air passages.[66] If quieting the mind on your own does not seem doable, then talk therapy could be a solution. Research has shown that cognitive behavioral therapy for people who have trouble sleeping helps to reduce sleep disturbances and occurrences of insomnia.[67]

Integrative health professionals have recommended natural over-the-counter sleep aids such as valerian root and melatonin for years as a temporary fix for sleep issues. On the flip side, there are also prescription options available. In 2012, 60 million prescriptions for sleeping pills in the United States, 43 million of which were for some form of zolpidem, which includes Ambien and Ambien CR,[68] were written. "All of the current (prescription sleep aids) on the market take a sledgehammer to specific receptors in the brain," says Dr. Robert McCarley, the head of psychiatry at Boston VA Medical Center and a professor of psychiatry at Harvard Medical School. "They have several negative side effects, ranging from disassociated states of consciousness to potential addiction. They also tend to lose their effectiveness over time."[69] Any drug that is taken for a drawn-out period of time can be tough for some people to give up. A specific side effect of many prescription sleep aids that may be experienced when you stop taking them is insomnia, which is worse than before you started taking the drug in the first place.[70]

It's clear that sleep deficiency can impact all areas of the body: learning, problem solving, decision-making, reaction time, trouble controlling emotions, and behavior. The way we feel when we're awake directly depends on how much high-quality sleep we were able to achieve the night before. Tonight, try and adjust your routine to accommodate some new positive sleep hygiene ideas and wake feeling refreshed and ready to conquer the day.

Think you have a sleep problem? Complete the checklist in the back of the book and discuss the answers with your doctor.

INTERVIEW: The importance of sleep with Dr. Ana C. Krieger, MD, MPH, associate professor of medicine, neurology, and genetic medicine at New York-Presbyterian Hospital/Weill Cornell Medical College

Much of the scientific evidence that revolves around sleep has only been brought to light in recent years. What sparked this interest in studying sleep and why did it take so long?

DR. ANA C. KRIEGER: Technological advances were key to the understanding of sleep and the development of sleep research. Since the discovery of electroencephalography (EEG) about 80 years ago, the field has grown exponentially, leading to the identification of sleep stages and the ability to record and monitor brain activity during sleep. The major jump in sleep research occurred after the description of sleep-related respiratory problems in the 1960s. Over the past 20 years, the field of sleep medicine has continued to rapidly expand and moved from obscurity to a well-known medical specialty.

What constitutes high-quality sleep and is there a way to make sure you get it?

DAK: Different layman's terms have been used to qualify sleep. Basically, the concept pertains to the fact that sleep is a dynamic process, constantly changing during the night in an organized and somewhat predictable fashion. Interruptions of the sleep cycle lead to fragmented sleep, which may be considered "low quality." Recent data suggest that the restorative functions of sleep are more effectively achieved when adequate or uninterrupted sleep is present, even for a shorter than ideal duration, as compared to longer durations of fragmented sleep, indicating that a "partial" rest is better than no rest at all. Ensuring a quiet and restful sleep period is a necessary step to achieve adequate sleep health in the population.

Does managing our energy with active rest or meditation provide the same benefits as sleep?

DAK: Quiet rest and meditation may allow the brain activity to change into similar patterns as the ones seen during the early stages of sleep. Despite providing some rest to the brain and the body, there is no evidence they can fully replace sleep.

Do seasonal changes affect our circadian rhythm or does our circadian rhythm stay relatively the same throughout the year?

DAK: The circadian rhythm in humans is well synchronized to the 24-hour clock due to environmental cues that help with entrainment. For people living close to the Equator, there are minimal seasonal changes in daylight or sleep duration throughout the year. However, this may be quite different in people living in extreme latitudes due to the very limited light exposure during the winter months. This effect on circadian rhythm is now being studied, and it may lead to significant seasonal variability not only in sleep duration but also in the body's physiology. It is important to note, however, that indoor shields and the use of artificial light can easily modulate the environmental exposure to natural light.

I've met people in the United States who sleep with their cellphone under their pillows, so they can wake up in the middle of the night and answer emails. How does one reprioritize sleep in the digital age?

DAK: The technological advances we have seen over the past few decades are fantastic and have led to amazing discoveries and developments in all fields. The critical point here is to make sure we identify smart and efficient ways to use technology. Being diligent about appropriately allocating time to important tasks is critical. In the same way that it is not productive to eat a meal while exercising, trying to work amidst sleep is not an effective use of our time for either task. A better understanding of the physiological needs of our body is quite important. Once people recognize factors that affect sleep, such as light and stimuli in this case, they would be better able to develop strategies to optimize sleep.

When I'm sick all I want to do is sleep. If I allow myself to take a sick day instead of fighting with my body to stay awake, I get better faster. Why is this?

DAK: One of the functions of sleep is to boost our immune response; therefore, a need for adequate rest during sickness will enhance the recovery process. Recent evidence also points to the fact that even the immune response to vaccines is higher in people that sleep well as compared to people that have inadequate sleep.

According to a 2000 study conducted by the *British Medical Journal*, going 24 hours without sleep equates one's performance level to having a blood alcohol content of 0.1%, legally drunk in the United States. Why is our government not doing more to educate people on not driving while tired?

DAK: This is about to change. Due to increased awareness of the potential harmful effects of sleep loss, several new campaigns have been initiated to educate the public and in particularly the youth on the dangers of driving when tired. Sleep research and education in high schools has also increased, and several professional groups and employers have implemented educational programs aiming to reduce sleep deprivation among professionals. This trend will continue to rapidly increase over the next few years.

If someone were to start changing their sleep hygiene tonight, where should they begin?

DAK: One of the most important aspects to ensure good sleep is to have a set routine. Keeping a regular bedtime and wake time every day is critical for adequate regulation of circadian rhythms, which dictate many functions of our body in a well-synchronized fashion, including hormone secretion and alertness, closely tied to our 24-hour clock. Our circadian rhythm doesn't distinguish weekday from weekends, so yes, a regular sleep time should be kept 7 days a week whenever possible.

3

GET FIT

Confession: I spent $5,315 working out last year. This crazy amount of money bought me 45 yoga classes, 60 strength and toning classes, and 90 trampoline cardio classes in New York City. But my fitness sessions were not limited to what I paid for. I also received complimentary workouts from wellness instructors who invited me to their classes, and I participated in all the fitness sessions on the wellness travel tours I led, which means the actual price tag for these sessions is probably triple.

So, why the heck am I willing to spend all this hard-earned cash on a fitness routine? I learned very quickly that in order to keep me motivated to work out, I needed to make an appointment for a set class time, one where I would lose money if I bailed. Working out alone gave me too many outs and excuses not to do it, and while losing money was not an option, it wasn't the only motivating factor; the classes had to excite me so I looked forward to attending. It took a lot of experimenting, but like Goldilocks, I finally found a formula that is just right for me. My current fitness routine stimulates me, keeps me happy (plus those around me), makes me feel good, and embraces me into a community. After more than 20 years of working out in my adult life trying to find a fitness routine that doesn't feel like a chore, I've finally found my jam.

Living in New York City, you tend to spend money just walking out the door. Yet balancing my fitness budget against my former way of living—paying to eat out daily (sometimes all 3 meals), after-work cocktails, weekly clothes shopping—I actually spend less per month now than I used to. Today, I eat out only a few times a month and rarely drink alcohol. I shop seasonally for fitness clothing, and I can't remember the last time I went to the pharmacy to pick up a prescription or even made a sick appointment to see the doctor. Plus, working out has become my therapy, a place to kick stress to the curb and literally get out of my head. I made the conscious decision to focus my spending on my fitness, and in exchange I am happier, healthier, and more prudent with my money than I used to be. Year after year, I am willing to spend this kind of money on my "get fit" routine because it provides me with more than just a healthy-looking body.

In prehistoric times, survival depended on our level of physical fitness. Scarce resources forced tribes to be nomadic in search of food and water. During the Neolithic agricultural revolution, inventions allowed us to stop roaming and stay put in order to cultivate food via farming, which required hard physical labor. As ancient civilizations grew and modern societies developed, hard labor tasks were eliminated. The Greeks and their medical practitioners developed movements set to music (gymnastics) in order to keep their bodies strong and minds healthy. As wealth grew for many during the Roman Empire, physical fitness levels started to change as material possession became more important to the upper class. This also meant more people spent more time indoors. The lavish lifestyle and excess of food for the rich developed the first foray into a sedentary lifestyle some 1,800 years ago. As the United States was settled and multiple cultures developed the land, physical fitness routines became a mesh of these traditions: gymnastics, calisthenics, swimming, running, walking, farming, and horseback riding. In the nineteenth century, as the first universities were established on the East Coast, intellect began to trump movement, which paved the way for our current routine: choosing inactivity over activity, a sedentary lifestyle.

PLEASE, DON'T TAKE A SEAT

> *A bear, however hard he tries, grows tubby without
> exercise.*[1]

> —A. A. Milne, *Teddy Bear*

Ouch. Do you feel a pain in your lower back? What about a strain in your neck? Is your mind wandering during the workday? Have you stretched your legs today or have you been sitting at your desk for the past six hours? Humans were born to be active, and too much time spent sitting in front of a computer, sitting in front of the television, sitting in cars, in trains, in buses, and on flights is causing our muscular and respiratory systems strain. Technological advances have forced us into a chair for hours at a time, creating a sedentary lifestyle. Our daily routines are putting us at greater risk of developing cardiovascular disease[2] and advancing the aging process,[3] while it restructures our musculoskeletal body, all because we have come to choose convenience over physical exertion.

"Sitting has become the smoking of our generation,"[4] declared Nilofer Merchant, a Fortune 500 consultant and author, in her 2013 TED Talk. And she's right. Our society has evolved to the point where almost everything is available with a click of a mouse or within driving distance. Why should we move in search of food, water, or entertainment when we can get everything we need delivered to our door 24/7? Sitting in the twenty-first century, especially at work where we spend the better part of our day, is the new normal.

Spending hours a day in a seated position pushes our bodies into an unnatural physical state. When seated, our frame tends to slump forward, curving the spine into a C shape. This puts uneven strain and pressure on the vertebrae, lumbar column, and the thoracic spine, which means some muscles get overworked while others suffer due to underworking. Because "dem bones" are all connected, this C curve allows the abs to go unused and enables the shoulders to collapse into a hunched position. Rounding out this C curve, the head hangs or juts forward, forcing the neck and trapezius muscles to support it, which is an extra 10 pounds of weight! Sit this way for hours every day and soon the body grows accustomed to the position, creating permanent imbalances which can lead to chronic lower back and neck pains.[5]

Internally, our lungs and pulmonary system also suffer from prolonged sitting. The C curve our body adapts is essentially bad posture, which restricts lung capacity[6] as we are unable to take full deep breaths. With the lungs incapable of fully expanding due to bad posture, blood flow is restricted, stymieing the amount of oxygen we intake. This causes brain fog or the inability to stay alert due to the reduced flow of blood and oxygen to the brain.[7]

Celebrity fitness trainer Harley Pasternak, who counts Jane Fonda, Halle Berry, and Lady Gaga as his clients, has made it his life's mission to get people up and moving throughout the day. He recently published an article titled "Even Physically Active Women Sit Too Much." In it, he cited a Northwestern University study, which revealed that people who work out 2.5 hours a week or about 20 minutes a day are still sitting more than they move.[8] This information may seem obvious when stated this way, but it is a clear reminder how much we sit each day and serves as a serious wakeup call: we simply spend too much time on our butts.

Having identified rising obesity rates as a continuous problem in developed countries, Dr. Melanie Luhrmann from the University of Royal Holloway in London hypothesized that our sedentary lifestyle may be the culprit. Her latest study focused on these rising rates and noted that over the last 30 years obesity rates have almost tripled, despite the fact that our caloric intake has fallen by about 20%.[9] A sedentary lifestyle has struck again.

Researchers at the University of Cambridge in the United Kingdom also became interested in the twenty-first century's collective lack of exercise and set out to study the long-term effects. Results from the 12-year study, which published in January 2015, concluded that all this sitting puts us at twice the risk of early death compared to obesity.[10] As scientific evidence continues to pour in, it is becoming clearer every day that getting up from our screens has never been more important to our life.

STEP AWAY FROM THE SCREEN

> *Physical inactivity should be recognized as a global pandemic and should be treated like any other infectious-disease pandemic would be.*[11]

—Dr. Harold W. Kohl

The Centers for Disease Control defines physical activity as "any bodily movement produced by the contraction of skeletal muscle that increases energy expenditure above a basal level."[12] As manufacturing jobs leave the United States and the commercial farming industry shrinks, our time spent at work moves from physically demanding professions to sitting behind computer screens, which leaves our leisure time hours as the only period to get active. Yet approximately 36% of adults in the United States do not engage in any physically active pursuits during leisure time.[13] This is costing us a pretty penny when it comes to our physical, mental, and emotional health and well-being.

Physical inactivity is the primary cause of many chronic diseases such as diabetes, stroke, arthritis, hypertension, heart disease, and cancer, all of which tangibly manifest in the body. In 2008, more than 5.3 million deaths worldwide were ascribed to physical inactivity in developed countries.[14] In the United States alone, healthcare expenditures attributed toward physical inactivity were upwards of $2.4 billion a year.[15] This same year the *Framingham Heart Study* introduced the concept of Heart Age, which revealed that average heart age for U.S. adults was significantly higher—between 5.4 and 7.8 years higher—than our chronological age.[16] All of this information is concrete scientific evidence that one would think would be a motivating factor to get everyone everywhere up and moving. Unfortunately, it is not.

I can tell you from my own experience that when I exercise I get sick less often and my stress levels are better managed. The endurance I've built in my cardiovascular and muscular system makes small tasks such as moving furniture, running to catch a bus, or carrying heavy groceries for blocks much easier. While these are easily identifiable improvements in my daily life, that's not all that happens to your body when you are able to commit to a routine fitness plan.

Are You More at Risk for Disease if You Don't Workout?

According to a 2015 article published in the *American Journal of Medicine*,[1] lack of physical activity in the United States accounts for the following:

- 22% of coronary heart disease
- 22% of colon cancer
- 18% of osteoporotic fractures
- 12% of diabetes and hypertension
- 5% of breast cancer

NOTE

1. Lewis, Steven and Charles H. Hennekens. "Regular Physical Activity: Forgotten Benefits," *The American Journal of Medicine*, February 2016. DOI: 10.1016/J.Amjmed.2015.07.016

Dr. Frank Booth, a prominent researcher and professor of biomedical sciences at the University of Missouri, points to a lack of physical activity as the primary cause for initiating 35 separate pathological and clinical conditions such as metabolic syndrome, obesity, insulin resistance, prediabetes, nonalcoholic liver disease, cardiovascular disease, impaired cognitive functions, bone and connective tissue disorders, cancer, reproductive diseases, and diseases of the digestive tract and kidney,[17] to name a few.

On its own, cardiovascular disease is the leading cause of deaths in both men and women in the United States. Each year, a quarter, or about 610,000, of the deaths in America are from heart disease.[18] Cardiovascular disease affects not only the heart but also the blood vessels. Those who do not exercise regularly have been shown to have higher rates of cardiovascular events, which lead to higher rates of death from those events.[19] As a preventative measure, exercise can thwart these incidents. If you have a hereditary condition, have been newly diagnosed with heart disease, or have just suffered a cardiac event, there is a silver lining. Studies have shown that patients who establish an exercise routine are able to return to work earlier and show faster quality of life improvements such as decreases in stress, less anxiety, and more self-confidence than those who do not exercise.[20]

One of the biggest benefits of exercise is that it normalizes your glucose, insulin, and leptin levels.[21] If you have diabetes or are at risk of developing diabetes, this makes regular physical activity your friend—maybe even your best friend. According to Dr. Booth, finding a daily physical activity routine if you have type 2 diabetes can actually reverse insulin resistance if your body is otherwise healthy.[22] While diabetes primarily affects the major organs of the bodily system, once you have the disease, your skeletal system is at risk too.

A recent study published in the *Bone Journal* looked at bone fractures in diabetics, a potentially life-threatening ailment. The research showed that one in six diabetics who suffered hip fractures died within one year.[23] Since physical inactivity is the primary cause of bone loss in weight-bearing bones in both diabetics and nondiabetics, the study concluded that improving bone health via exercise will reduce the risk of fractures and therefore the risk of death related to those fractures.[24] If you do not have diabetes, don't make the mistake of thinking bone loss doesn't apply to you. Peak bone density in healthy adults is achieved at around age 30; from here this density slowly starts to decline, ultimately leading to osteoporosis.[25] Working out improves overall posture, joints, and muscle mass, as well as bone density.

If you've ever been on crutches, had surgery that left a part of your body immobile, or have spent time in a wheelchair, you may have joked about how it turned you into an "old man" once you were able to free yourself of those devices. Turns out it's actually not a joke. A study undertaken at the University of Copenhagen found that younger people around 23 years of age who went two weeks without using their legs lost one-third of their muscular strength, leaving their bodies on par with a person 40 to 50 years their senior.[26]

Finding and sustaining a regular exercise routine isn't just beneficial to those who have contracted or are at higher risk of contracting a physical life-threatening disease; if you feel good now and have a clean bill of health, your internal systems will still benefit from the activity and keep you on a healthy path. Doctors at the Mayo Clinic in Minnesota tell us that exercise reduces LDL or "bad" cholesterol and can raise the HDL or "good" cholesterol in your bloodstream,[27] which is something everyone can relate to and benefit from.

Weight loss is probably the most common reason that people turn to exercise, and I hate to break it to you, but exercise alone is not going to keep the pounds off long-term. Eric Ravussin, a weight loss expert and professor at the Pennington Biomedical Research Center in Baton Rouge, Louisiana, told *The New York Times Magazine*: "In general, exercise by itself is pretty useless for weight loss. It's especially useless because people often end up consuming more calories when they exercise."[28]

But don't let this discourage you, as consistent exercise does prevent excess weight gain and helps to decrease the rate of regain if you've been able to lose weight in the first place.[29] When you develop a regular fitness routine, you may see a spike in your hunger levels immediately, but over time your biological need to eat more is reduced as exercise establishes a new homeostasis. Why is this? Exercise remodels the metabolic pathways of the body and changes the way it stores and utilizes food intake. When you exercise, your body tends to burn fat immediately after you eat, whereas a sedentary person burns carbohydrates instead and stores the fat to be used at a later date.[30]

Creating and maintaining a realistic and regular physical fitness routine is not an easy feat, but it is the common denominator in multiple studies which show maintained weight loss. I-Min Lee, a researcher at the Harvard Medical School, looked at weight change histories in more than 30,000 women. Publishing her findings in the *Journal of the American Medical Association*,[31] Lee showed that women who participated in nonstrenuous exercise almost every day not only gained far less weight than women who did not have a consistent fitness routine, but that they were able to maintain their body size over the years.

Movement is at the core of the wellness lifestyle. While you may start down a fitness path in order to lose or maintain weight, lower cholesterol, improve cardio function, or counteract the effects of sitting all day, it's the instant gratification that keeps us coming back day in and day out. Exercise

Easy Ways to Add Physical Activity to Your Life Starting Now

- **Make it a game**—Invest in wearable tech that shows your steps or sign up for a fun run. By taking the focus off the exercise itself and instead honing in on setting and reaching a goal, meeting that goal will be enjoyable instead of a chore.
- **Take the stairs**—This low-impact aerobic exercise is easy, safe, and accessible. Have your office building open the stairwell or stop by the high school stadium on your way home from work. As a full body movement, climbing the stairs exercises your heart, calves, quadriceps, and glutes while it releases endorphins and burns calories.
- **Turn up the music**—Tap your toes, shake your hips, and move your booty along to the music while you get dressed in the morning or do the dishes at night. You'll increase your aerobic fitness and put a smile on your face.
- **Ditch your car**—Instead of driving down the road to the store, lace up your sneakers or hop on a bike to run your errands. If leaving your car behind is not an option, then park a few blocks from your final destination and hoof it.

heightens mood and gives a huge self-confidence booster, while at the same time it's helping relieve stress and anxiety. If you've ever experienced a runner's high, then you know: that is some powerful stuff.

When he was interviewed for a cover story on the benefits of exercise for mental health, Michael Otto, a professor of psychology at Boston University, told the American Psychological Association: "The link between exercise and mood is pretty strong. Usually within five minutes after moderate exercise you get a mood-enhancement effect."[32] Ohio-based therapist Jennifer Carter regularly schedules her client sessions outdoors in the form of a walk,[33] and clinical psychologist Dr. James Blumenthal states that exercise is not only important for treating depression, but is also important for preventing relapses.[34] Noticing a pattern here?

When you go for a run or a brisk walk through the park, when you set up your yoga mat or hit the gym to lift weights, you are producing endorphins. These natural painkillers improve our ability to deal with stress, anxiety, and depression. Plus, they make us feel really good. Exercise forces the body's physiological systems to communicate closely with each other: the respiratory system talks to the nervous system; the cardiovascular system speaks to the renal system. This full body exchange enables you to be more efficient at squashing stress and anxiety when they arise.

According to the Anxiety and Depression Association of America, these effects may be short term, but they can deliver several hours of relief post-workout as opposed to just popping a pill to deal with your symptoms.[35] A regular sweaty, heart-pumping workout routine for people who are prone to anxiety might help in preventing attacks from happening in the first place. Take high-intensity interval training (HIIT), an exercise approach that intersperses short periods of intense anaerobic moves with longer aerobic recovery periods (think one minute of sprinting into a four-minute jog repeated over the course of 30 minutes) as an example. HIIT is recommended for patients with chronic heart failure in order to strength the heart muscle,[36] but it has also been clinically shown to reduce anxiety sensitivity.[37]

When participating in HIIT, you are exposing your body to the same physical reactions that an anxiety attack creates: increasing your oxygen uptake, activating your fight-or-flight response, and elevating your heart rate. But you are doing this in a controlled setting where you can learn to regulate your breath between the bouts of intensive activity. Soon enough, the body starts to associate these symptoms with a safe place that you can control, not a danger zone.

Lack of physical activity is also attributed to causing up to 1/3 of the reported cases of depression.[38] Research suggests that by increasing serotonin, the neurotransmitter targeted by antidepressants, through exercise, you can actually prevent 20–30% of these reported cases.[39] If the idea of jumping out of bed to participate in some high-intensity exercise makes you want to pull the covers over your head instead, consider yoga. Yoga has shown acute benefits for people with depression. Practicing

Let's Move

With only 1/4 of kids in the United States getting the recommended daily amount of physical activity, try these simple suggestions to get them moving now and help them adapt physical fitness into their daily routine.

- **Make it a game**—Adults are not the only ones who enjoy games. The current generation is being raised on gamification, so find a way to make it fun so they stick with it, or join them outdoors for some Pokémon Go.
- **Tell them it'll make math easier**—Exercise has been linked to thinner gray matter and better math skills.
- **Talk about getting a bigger brain**—Kids who are fit tend to have a larger hippocampus, which allows them to perform better in tests at school.
- **Lead by example**—Don't pressure your kids to join you, but set a good example. Kids who make their own decisions about exercise typically identify as "exercise people."

yoga influences neurotransmitters, inflammation, and oxidative stress in a way that is very similar to antidepressants and psychotherapy.[40] With over 21 million adults in the United States practicing yoga,[41] it is easy to find a class and style that appeals to your ideal "get fit" program.

Tackling the physical body as well as our emotional and mental states are all huge benefits of fitness, but can working out also make us smarter? Our brains need oxygen and blood to function. When increasing these essentials to the brain, it benefits us almost immediately with better real-time function. When regularly increasing that flow, the brain grows new brain cells which boost memory and learning.[42] This happens because the brain-derived neurotrophic factor (BDNF) gene, the gene responsible for instructing the brain to make a protein that promotes nerve cell survival and their connections within our brain, responds to exercise and improves these functions.

As we age our hippocampus, the part of our brain where we store memory shrinks. The brain's hippocampal plasticity is dependent on BDNF processing. Exercise triggers BDNF stimulation, improving our cognitive function and slowing the progression of Alzheimer's disease[43] as well as decreasing the risk of dementia.[44] While a single session of exercise does nothing to increase memory function, a 4-week study conducted at Dartmouth College in New Hampshire found that regular aerobic fitness enhances object recognition memory,[45] or the brain's ability to retrieve details associated with a previous experience. Additionally, a Scottish study,[46] along with a separate Beckman Institute study,[47] concluded that people who exercise have larger brains where white matter, the part of the brain that acts as a relay to send communication throughout all parts of the brain, is more compact and prone to less shrinkage.

Exercise will also improve your sleep and your sex life. Long-term moderate physical activity improves your sleep quality almost 20%,[48] while it leaves you feeling better rested in the morning. When you are better rested, your quality of life improves because you're not constantly battling your body to stay awake. Now that you have some extra awake hours, you can spend that time in bed enjoying your sex life instead of sleeping. Regular physical activity can lead to enhanced arousal in women,[49] and men who exercise are less likely to experience problems with erectile dysfunction.[50] Often the more time we devote to our fitness, the happier we are with our physical appearance, which leads us to feeling sexier in the bedroom.

Clearly, it is important to find ways to stay active. A 20-minute brisk walk each day, which burns between 90 and 110 calories, moves you from the inactive to moderately inactive fitness category, reducing risk of premature death by 16–30%.[51] And it's never too late to start! Dr. Kirk Erickson, a psychology professor at the University of Pittsburgh, found that when sedentary adults, 65+, started walking for their workouts, they showed improved memory and increases in volume in the hippocampus,[52] leading to better problem-solving skills.

When we forgo physical activity, we put ourselves at risk of contracting any number of chronic physical diseases, ones that are slow in their progress, possibly decades in the making. Yet once these diseases take hold, they are lengthy in their continuance

and very hard to get rid of, which makes the argument for
starting preventative measures now even more enticing.

MEET ME FOR A SWEAT SESH

*So many people spend their health gaining wealth,
and then have to spend their wealth to regain their
health.*[53]

—A. J. Reb Materi

The question really becomes, with the amount of hours you
spend in the office, commuting to the office, traveling for the
office, entertaining clients, and participating in after work
office activities, who really has time to fit in exercise? It is this
frustration that has given rise to the popularity of working out
at work or during work hours, coining the term "sweatworking."

Sweatworking is holding a lunch meeting over a walk in the
park, scheduling client face-time into a bootcamp class at 5pm or
swapping out the next boozy office holiday party to gather the
team in a cycling studio. These sweat sessions have been sweeping
Wall Street, where expensive entertaining and playing just as
hard as you work is par for the course. John Abularrage, head
of the brokerage firm Tullett Prebon, told *Bloomberg Business*,
"When there's a lot of entertaining to do for your job, you can get
out of shape pretty quickly. Some clients are more eager than you
would imagine to trade a heavy dinner or drinks for a workout."[54]

Sweatworking may be becoming an increasingly popular
and accepted way of connecting with people outside of a traditional office setting, but what makes the case to bring the boss
or the head office on board? Increased productivity. A study
published in the *International Journal of Workplace Health and
Management* reported that 72% of people see improvements in
their time management, 74% manage their workload better, and
79% are more focused in the office on days that they exercise
compared to days when they don't.[55]

At the University of Bristol in the United Kingdom, an
exercise-at-work study was conducted to examine the effects on

Sweatworking 101

Ready to trade in that steak dinner for a sweat session? Here are some guidelines to follow, so that the experience is an enjoyable one for everyone.

- **Don't make this your first in-person meeting**—Get to know your client or coworker a little before you suggest sweatworking. The idea of taking business out of the office might be uncomfortable for some, so do not start your relationship in the locker room.
- **Let the client pick the workout**—You might love yoga, they might prefer spinning. As the one asking for the meeting, put your client at ease by letting them pick an environment they feel comfortable in. Who knows, you might even find your new obsession.
- **Head to different areas of the locker room**—Being naked around someone you see regularly in a business setting is just plain uncomfortable. Skip the headache and make a beeline for some privacy.
- **Don't wear your smelly sweats**—You may be trading your suit for workout gear, but you are not at home. Come prepared to this meeting like you would any other. With so many stylish fitness options to sweat in these days, make sure you are presentable.
- **Make sweatworking a company event**—If the idea of a one-on-one session is still too awkward, think about renting out a private room or studio for both coworkers and clients. Turn your next cocktail party into a healthier version with a little sweat followed by smoothies.

employee productivity. In addition to enhanced mood, tolerance, and resilience toward coworkers, the results revealed that workers who exercised held a competitive advantage and had increased motivation during working hours.[56] Jo Coulson, research associate on the study, says the results showed that "workers performed significantly better on exercise days"[57] across all three areas that the study measured: mental interpersonal (language and math skills), output or productivity, and time demands.

On days you are able to fit in a workout, don't you feel more accomplished? It's no coincidence that sweating it out before you sit for long periods of time makes you calmer and better equipped to handle anything that comes your way. Still don't feel comfortable with the thought of getting sweaty next to someone you don't know that well? Think of these sweat sessions as the new golfing.

Deals used to be done primarily by men on the back nine. Now companies are using sweatworking to level the playing field, allowing everyone the opportunity to bond with clients and close a deal. With entertainment budgets shrinking due to overall budget cuts, these sessions are even being used to boost creativity by following them with a brainstorming meeting.

Let's face it: there are not enough hours in the day to do everything, so why not get a two for one? Sweatworking increases your work productivity while allowing you to meet your personal fitness goals. Added bonus: if you're getting to put these pricy workouts on the company card, it means you are saving yourself money and the company in future healthcare costs down the road. These days, with the lines between work time and personal time being blurred anyway, it might as well be used to everyone's advantage.

LET'S GET PHYSICAL

> *Instagram feeds the enthusiasm for fitness and wellness because we share workouts, yoga poses, gorgeous salads and sexy smoothies. And that encourages other people to try it.*[58]
>
> —Well+Good founders
> Alexia Brue and Melisse Gelula

Working out is definitely the "it item" of the decade. Writer Marisa Meltzer, in her article "Why Fitness Classes are Making You Go Broke," wrote: "The height of opulence, especially in warm, fit cities, is being rich enough not to work so you can spend all of your time perfecting your body."[59] This might explain the drive, the need, or even the rationalization as to why some of the fitness-obsessed set are willing to shell out $37 for a 45-minute spin class or pay double to circumvent the waitlists of popular studios. Yet most people do not find themselves in this situation and instead have to look at their overall living expenses to figure out how to make it all work.

Swapping dinner and drinks at a trendy restaurant for a workout or asking for a fitness package to a favorite studio for a birthday gift are ways that responsible spenders have found to keep their costs down. There are also plenty of free or low-cost options, such as online apps or "first class free" offers from gyms and boutique studios that can be interspersed between paid sessions. The old school option of climbing stairs is another great way to get in cardio for free, even at work. "Stair climbing will give you a little more bang for your buck because of the vertical component, allowing you to burn more calories for the same amount of time [as jogging or cycling],"[60] says Cedric Bryant, chief science officer for the American Council on Exercise.

Are you one of the 80 million early adopters who sported a wearable in 2015?[61] Be it smart watch or fitness tracker, wearable technology is having a moment. Being able to measure yourself against a fixed goal pushes you toward success and shows in actual data points what you've achieved. This quantifiable data is great for people who want this type of engagement.

Once dismissed as gimmicks, wearable fitness trackers reached an estimated $7 billion in sales in 2015[62] and are poised to top more than 214 million users by 2019.[63] In June 2015, Fitbit's IPO closed at 52% higher than it opened,[64] proving the growth potential and staying power in this new technology sector. And while 75% of consumers say they'll be purchasing a wearable device in the next five years,[65] there is still a lot of work to be done when it comes to the precision of the data the devices deliver.

In the first study to compare the accuracy of different activity monitors, the Department of Kinesiology at Iowa State University tracked how popular wearables measure daily activity in everything from caloric expenditure to improving overall health. The data revealed that, while all the 2015 devices measured caloric consumption reasonably accurately, specific activities had margins of error, leading researchers to rate overall

Pricey Workout Hacks

Millennials are the generation that has truly been raised on wellness, yet most of them are not yet making enough to cover the cost of a pricy fitness regime. Here are some cost-effective ways they are sweating it out, which might be fun for you to try.

- **Post about it**—Just search Instagram for the #fitspo (that's fitness inspiration to you) hashtag to discover free new fitness moves to try or post about your own.
- **Join a tribe**—There are a plethora of online communities you can connect to that will keep you motivated and even offer meet ups so you can work out together for free.
- **YouTube it**—Many popular fitness instructors have YouTube channels that offer free content, which allows you to sweat along in your own home.
- **Put a Fitbit on it**—Millennials are leaders in the wearable tech industry. Find a gadget that works for you and find fun ways to accomplish your steps daily.
- **Change your mindset**—This generation started their wellness routines as kids and while that may not be the case for anyone 34 and above, adopt their outlook: wellness is not just about being fit, it's about being healthy.

error margins between 16.8% with the Fitbit Flex and up to 30.4% with the Misfit Shine (a tracker big in the Asian market).[66]

But the real question is: do users care if the data is accurate? According to Goldman Sachs' 2015 report, "Millennials, Coming of Age," this generation, the largest in history with the most spending power, see wellness as an active pursuit, and using wearable technology to push themselves to exercise more helps to shape how they curate their lifestyle.[67] As investment climbs and technology develops, fitness trackers will become more accurate and consumption will continue to increase.

Whether you're tracking fitness stats for your own pleasure or doing it in order to share your #fitspo with the world, it's clear we've seen just the tip of the iceberg, as wearables continue to emerge. Melisse Gelula and Alexia Brue, founders of online wellness magazine Well+Good, feel their readers have a healthy approach: "While it's certainly not mandatory for a workout, tech devices make staying active really fun and engaging."[68]

Modern medicine has helped our society cure serious infectious diseases with vaccines and antibiotics. We now live longer, healthier, more productive lives because of it. Today, most people die of a chronic disease—heart disease, cancer, or diabetes among them, all of which can be prevented or managed by committing to a get fit routine. For those who have already found their groove, fitness has been used to battle stress, anxiety, and depression. Oftentimes, purchasing a gym membership is less expensive than paying for therapy and the medication that may come along with it.

Using fitness to extend the quality of our lives and enhance our productivity at work makes for a good argument. So stop what you're doing right now—drop and give me five. Or go walk around the block. Or call up your coworker and change tonight's dinner into a sweat session. However you choose to add fitness to your life today, you'll feel better about it and yourself tomorrow.

INTERVIEW: Fitness and self-care with Alexia Brue and Melisse Gelula, founders of Well+Good, a premier lifestyle and news publication devoted to wellness

Being healthy has taken on a totally new meaning in the last 10 years; it is no longer just about your body being free of disease. How would you explain today's definition of health, and what areas of a person does it address?

Well+Good: There's definitely a broad spectrum in terms of how different people define health! At Well+Good, we take it to mean living your life while adding healthy things to it that give you balance, happiness, and great nutrition. In other words, are you actively adding things to your life that are healthy? That's the lifestyle approach we encourage. Good health is something people can pursue through working out or doing yoga, adding more kale salads to your diet or blending green, swapping current beauty products for cleaner ones, or getting into alternative therapies like naturopathy and acupuncture that help you deal with stress. It's about cultivating healthy relationships with these things in your own way. We encourage our readers to find their own recipe for their most vital health. It's not about dropping 5 pounds in 5 days, or melting fat, or flat abs, or what have you. The wellness revolution is about adding positive things to your life.

The wellness revolution is now being introduced to younger generations. In fact, yoga and meditation is being taught in the schools, and some new parents are making baby food instead of buying it. Was there a tipping point that started this revolution or was it a gradual shift?

W+G: We believe it was a gradual shift, with certain catalyzing moments. Obviously, there have always been people who prioritized wellness, but previously that lifestyle was seen as more fringe or alternative. To your example, making baby food was seen as "hippy-ish" (for lack of a better word), but now it's totally mainstream. Doing yoga used to be "alternative" or New Agey, and now over 21 million people in the United States practice it. Few people used to care about what was in their skincare and makeup, and now natural is the fastest growing segment in the beauty space. Across the board, it's now easier than ever to make healthy choices: more healthy food options on the go, more workout options, etc. It's incredibly exciting that this lifestyle is available to so many people.

A plethora of articles have been published recently about business meetings moving into the gym. When and why did this start to happen, and are people really OK breaking a sweat next to a potential client or coworkers?

W+G: Client entertaining is a big part of the job in many fields and it often happens in restaurants (often unhealthy ones) and over drinks. Many people started to recognize the toll this took on their health. When SoulCycle burst on the scene in 2006, it had all the cache of a club, and healthy-leaning account managers realized they could swap drinks for a SoulCycle class and smoothie. Breakfast and sweatworking, a term now in common use that we've written about and referenced a lot, grew from there. Of course, not everyone is comfortable dripping sweat next to potential clients, but more and more people are, and classes like indoor cycling in a dark room and yoga that's not too sweaty are good starter sweatworking sessions.

Is New York City leading the wellness charge with new fitness studios, wellness centers, a bike share program, and the "greening" of the city, or are other U.S. cities committing to residents, health, and wellness?

W+G: We published four Healthy City Guides (Boston, Chicago, Los Angeles, and San Francisco) in 2015. In all these cities, there's a healthy living revolution happening just like in New York City over the past five years. Juice bars, healthy restaurants, fitness, and yoga studios are opening at fast clips. Los Angeles has always had a robust wellness scene, particularly with juicing and yoga. (But we'd say it's not been as commercial as New York City, since hiking and surfing aren't brick-and-mortar experiences.) Natural beauty stores are now opening across the country, too, but we don't have many in New York City because of the cost of real estate.

Well+Good NYC published an article in 2013 about the skyrocketing price of boutique fitness classes, which can get up to $40/per class. Why are people willing to pay this kind of money and does it come at a sacrifice?

W+G: Many people who used to meet for drinks or dinner after work with friends now have shifted spending to fitness and wellness. Working out is the current way we socialize. Studios prioritize the entertainment factor with things such as great lighting, sound systems, and DJs. Places like Barry's Bootcamp, SoulCycle, and Barre3 create a "this is the place to be" vibe. The caliber of instruction is high and specialized, and teachers are recruited and trained for their charisma as much as their fitness skill. Customer service and amenities are high, too. This says that people don't mind spending money on things that are actually enriching to them. We call it "life-enhancing consumerism."

Life-enhancing consumerism feels more justifiable, emotionally fulfilling, and psychologically powerful than collecting $600 shoes a la Carrie Bradshaw. In the *Sex and the City* era, people were obsessed with the it bag and the it shoes; these days, working out at SoulCycle and walking around with green juice are the cultural aspirations. It's way healthier and way more attainable than what came before in terms of cultural obsessions.

4

GET ZEN

"Ohmmmmm. Ohmmmmm. Ohmmmmm." Cross-legged on a floor cushion in a dimly lit room at 7am, I carefully winked one eye open to see if anyone else was slumped over and snoring. Having just sat through a 45-minute meditation session, I wasn't sure if any of it took. My lower extremities were completely asleep, and just three minutes ago, I was pretty sure the rest of me was, too.

Our meditation guide, a twenty-something in a plaid shirt with soulful eyes shaded by heavy-framed dark glasses, asked us to open our eyes and share our experience. Thankfully, this took another 10 minutes, as I knew if I tried to get up while my legs were coursing with pins and needles, I would have hobbled around bent over like someone twice my age (I was 30) and given away the fact that I was a meditation novice.

I found myself in this donation session early one winter morning in New York's East Village because I was stressed out, burnt out, and heading into the scariest moment of my life: quitting my secure, well-paying job (with stellar healthcare coverage) to launch a company in an industry I knew absolutely nothing about.

Ending up in this small room was not that much of a leap for me. I'd practiced yoga for over 10 years at that point and was very aware of talk around meditation and its anecdotal benefits. Yet up until this point, the yoga I had been practicing focused on the asana, or exercise benefits, with only a small amount of chanting and breathing exercises sprinkled throughout. Sitting down for the sole purpose of clearing my mind was a first.

With a totally new life on the horizon—that of an entrepreneur, no less—just thinking about all the new challenges I would face overwhelmed me: How would I establish myself? Would I run out of money? What if I failed? These paralyzing questions and creeping doubts about my ability to run a successful company would (and sometimes still do) keep me up at night. It was time for me to add to my toolbox and find a way to breathe again without gasping.

THE RISE OF STRESS

> *When we get too busy and flustered we often forget*
> *to breathe and just be in the moment.*[1]

> —Dr. Frank Lipman

Since the 1970s, life expectancy in the United States has risen by more than 10 years due to major advances in healthcare. Today, on average, we live to 79 years of age.[2] Compare this number against the 2015 official retirement age—set by the U.S. government—of 66, and this leaves most of us with an average of 13 years to live off the wealth we've amassed during our 40+ years in the workforce.

Yet these numbers do not take into account the life we actually live. People get laid off, we spend our life savings putting our children through college, our parents or partners get unexpectedly sick; virtually anything can happen, while the cost of living soars around us and our own health declines as we age. Add in work stress, which has increased over the preceding decade due to our connectivity, availability, and workload increases, and it's enough to send anyone into panic mode. It is no wonder that stress levels are rising at alarming rates.

One of our biggest sources of stress is the constant connection we have to everything at all times through our digital devices: iPhone, iPad, laptop, AppleTV, Amazon Prime, Netflix, Hulu—I could go on. This endless interaction from the touch of

Is Job Stress Making You an Emotional Mess?

According to statistics gathered by the *American Institute of Stress*,[1] today's office environments are hotbeds of stress no matter the industry.

- 25% of people view their jobs as the number one stressor in their lives.
- 25% have felt like screaming or shouting because of job stress.
- 19%, or almost 1 in 5, have quit a previous position because of job stress.
- 1 in 4 have been driven to tears because of workplace stress.
- 10% are concerned about an individual at work they fear could become violent.

NOTE

1. American Institute of Stress, "Workplace Stress," http://www.cdc.gov/niosh/pdfs/87-111.pdf

a button on the couch or from the bed is responsible for sending our overworked adrenals and stress hormones into shock, contributing to health problems like obesity and exhaustion at any age.

The National Institute of Mental Health tells us that 40 million American adults[3] are affected by anxiety disorders. This is 18% of our population who at any given time are walking around suffering the physical manifestations of these issues such as depression, migraines, high blood pressure, heart disease, digestive disorders, and chronic pain. The Centers for Disease Control and Prevention (CDC) estimates that 75% of healthcare is spent on preventable chronic illness brought on, in part, by stress.[4]

Herbert Benson, founder of the Mind/Body Medical Institute in Massachusetts and author of the best-selling book *The Relaxation Response*, says, "Stress is a physiological response to any change, whether good or bad, that alerts the adaptive fight-or-flight response in the brain and the body. Good stress, also called 'eustress,' gives us energy and motivates us to strive and produce."[5] Yet we go through our days completely over-loaded and distracted, leaving our brain in a constant state of fight-or-flight because chronic stress and anxiety never let us resolve any of these issues.

The evolutionary purpose of our fight-or-flight response, a bodily reaction to the threat of survival, has morphed into a con-stant state of agitation and arousal leading to sustained mental anxiety that reveals itself in our physical health. Our body reacts to today's stress like it did to yesterday's equivalent: fear. We continuously push ourselves into survival mode, preventing any hope of learning, understanding, and emotionally coping.

It's clear we are trying to do too much. Today's social norms expect us to cram 18 hours of work into 10-hour workdays, eat healthy, exercise at least three times a week, run errands, raise our children, and relax without electronic devices before we get a good night's sleep. It's no wonder that the idea of multitasking was created. How the heck are we supposed to live like this day in and day out?

A few years ago, it was a badge of honor to claim you were a great multitasker, able to juggle multiple projects with speed and efficiency while still attending to your email and daily work duties. Apparently, we all had the wrong idea. A 2011 study out of the University of California, San Francisco, proved that multitasking negatively affects our short-term memory as a result of the interaction between attention and memory.[6] The study went on to reveal that as we age, our ability to ignore distraction diminishes. The switching back and forth between tasks without being fully engaged in either of them actually hurts our overall work productivity, and it takes us more time to get less done.

With all these circuit overloads, we are bound to blow a fuse, or worse yet, completely burn out at some point. Harvard psy-chiatrist and author Edward Hallowell agrees and claims the brain overload caused by our current working environments starts to manifest in physical symptoms such as distraction, inner frenzy, and impatience. When experiencing what he calls the attention deficit trait (ADT), people have trouble staying organized, setting priorities, and managing their time.[7]

Attention Deficit Trait

If you hold any kind of management position where you put out fires every day, feel increasingly hurried and curt toward your staff, or feel like you barely have time to focus on your own work, you may be developing ADT (Attention Deficit Trait). Discovered by Harvard psychiatrist Dr. Edward Hallowell, ADT appears to have the same symptoms as ADHD (Attention Deficit Hyperactivity Disorder), but the symptoms disappear when you are able to take a long break from your workload—for example, by going on vacation. If you are affected by ADT, try these simple steps now to get a handle on your workday:

- **Request a face-to-face meeting**—Create an emotional connection with your staff instead of trying to solve a problem over email.
- **Develop an organized work strategy**—Oftentimes the big picture overwhelms us. Try breaking down a project into smaller more manageable tasks and turn off your email when you sit down to work on them.
- **Schedule in a portion of your day for nothing**—Leave 30 minutes of your day open to thinking or planning. If the thought of this creates more stress, instead fill in this time with a mundane task (filing, reorganizing your bookshelf) and give your brain time to shut down. Eventually, you'll learn to relax enough to be open to big ideas.
- **Rearrange the setup of your workspace**—Move your desk to face a wall, open the blinds to let in more natural light, or put in headphones to drown out ambient noise. Sometimes a physical change can prompt a mental one.

Asking our brains to track all this data is like playing with a house of cards—adding one more piece to the pile will eventually make the entire system collapse. Our ability to creatively solve problems in this state starts to decline and our mistakes increase. Hallowell and his research tell us that employees who suffer from ADT will underachieve, create clutter, cut corners, and squander their brainpower. His examination of current companies show that when management continues to increase demands without providing relief, they end up creating a toxic, high-pressure environment that leads to a high rate of employee illness and turnover.[8]

If you are an employee who ties their self-worth and ideas of success to job achievements, this kind of high-pressured environment can begin to activate a negative stress cycle and lead to anxiety disorders and physical ailments such as cardiovascular disease.[9] The on-the-job stresses of long hours, perception of unfairness, and job insecurity build up over the years, spilling out into all areas of our lives. Under this kind of chronic stress, we shift into crisis mode, which compromises our ability to think clearly and make positive decisions for ourselves. The fight-or-flight survival symptoms our body creates in reaction to stress spill over into the workplace in the form of anxiety, missed deadlines, presenteeism, absenteeism, lateness, issues with your coworkers, and may even lead to you quitting your job—sound familiar?

THE WESTERN ORIGINS OF ZEN

> *I wouldn't stick my neck out this far (in support of meditation) if I didn't think **THIS** was the thing that could really shift the country.*[10]
>
> —U.S. Congressman Tim Ryan

So how did we get here? If stress really is the underlying cause of many of our physical and mental health ailments today, why are we not addressing it as a nation? Where are the TV commercials and print ads advocating for a national "stop and smell the roses" campaign or a public holiday that tells us to sit down and do nothing? While this has yet to materialize (and may never happen), in the past decade there has been a more conscious shift toward the intention of stress reduction. More bankers and business people are forgoing the drug- and alcohol-fueled nights of yore and are looking for healthier relaxation solutions that allow us to live our 10 additional years of longevity with a higher quality.

In the 1960s, U.S. immigration laws were loosened and our borders opened to various cultures from around the world. Buddhist Monks soon flocked to the West to teach Eastern philosophy throughout our storied institutions of higher education. By the 1970s, Buddhist practices had spread throughout the United States, and Naropa University, a four-year Buddhist college in Boulder, Colorado, was established.

During this movement, scientist Jon Kabat-Zinn was introduced to the Buddhist practice of meditation while working toward his molecular biology degree at MIT. Kabat-Zinn was so taken with this concept and how it could apply to anyone's life regardless of religious beliefs that he created a program called Mindfulness-Based Stress Reduction (MBSR).

As Kabat-Zinn delved deeper into the scientific benefits of mindfulness throughout the 1980s, he conducted clinical trials that showed MBSR training was successful in the treatment of chronic pain.[11] In the early 1990s, he published his first instructional book: a how-to for starting your own MBSR practice at home. Suddenly, the Public Broadcasting System (PBS) took notice and featured him on their program. MBSR clinics began opening in hospitals, while Dr. Kabat-Zinn spread the healing benefits of this practice across the nation through workshops and lecture. He is now known as *the* mindfulness research pioneer.

As fervor over Y2K built at the end of the last century, we as a society started to question the pace and rat race in which many of us worked. Ironically, we turned toward technology in search of answers and were collectively introduced to mindfulness practice by way of the Internet. At this point in the West, the mindfulness practice had started to leave its Buddhist association behind, as our analytic culture emphasized the health and scientific benefits instead.

Today, mindfulness is having its moment in the sun. In February 2014, *Time Magazine*'s cover read: "The Mindful Revolution." On the last day of 2014, *New Republic*'s front-page headline screamed, "How 2014 Became the Year of Mindfulness." You can't open a business publication today without reading how CEOs such as Mark Bertolini of Aetna, Toney Hsieh of Zappos, and the late Steve Jobs profess their success to meditation. Prior to his retirement, you could find Kobe Bryant meditating courtside, and Jerry Seinfeld has been known to repeat his personal mantra between takes on set. Lifestyle gurus from Oprah Winfrey to Deepak Chopra to Arianna Huffington have all created programs to help us sit and be mindful.

How did this happen? Why is mindfulness now the buzzword on everyone's lips? In the last 30 years alone, the West has produced 1,300 studies on meditation, and it seems people are finally taking notice. Smartphone apps dedicated to mindfulness are released daily, and people no longer have to sneak off during lunch to find their Zen, as there is a meditation room near the espresso machine. So what is it exactly that people are after, and how does mindfulness achieve this?

WHAT IS MINDFULNESS, AND HOW DO WE GET SOME?

At the end of the day, I can end up just totally wacky, because I've made mountains out of molehills. With meditation, I can keep them as molehills.[12]

—Ringo Starr

Most people who have no experience with mindfulness immediately conjure up an image of a serene being sitting on the floor, legs twisted at odds angles, meditating or chanting. And while that is how this chapter began, it is by no means the only form, or the right form.

The practice of mindfulness simply means focusing your attention on one thing fully for one moment. While there is a lot of weighty meaning packed into that sentence, you can be yourself in the "here and now" during any one of your daily activities like jogging, doing the dishes, eating a meal in silence, or by sitting in a formal meditation practice for just 15 minutes a day. This is where you can find your less stressed, more Zen "you." While options often seem limitless, there are essentially two main mindfulness techniques you can apply in your everyday life:

Mindful or focused-attention meditation is concentrating on the breath or the body or a phrase in a nonjudgmental way. With time, patience, and practice, you begin to build these moments into minutes. These accumulated bits of time start allowing you to experience life more fully, changing your relationship with the world and your perceived problems. A mindful state allows you to cultivate your personal strengths and reverse your self-limiting thoughts and behavior.

Open-monitoring meditation is the other often-studied form of meditation. This form does not request present-centered awareness, but instead asks practitioners to sit in observation. Notice your body, your breath, and your mind without reacting. This form of meditation asks that you fully experience whatever arises, thoughts and feelings, without labeling, judging, or analyzing them.

Dr. Miles Neale, a New York-based Buddhist psychotherapist, says that any kind of mindfulness practice calms us down and short circuits our reactive behavior. "Our experience is mainly based on associations, wired in by past experience, and our reactions are largely automatic. We are neither free to experience reality clearly in real time, nor free to choose how to respond. We are slaves to prefab interpretations and reactions, which not only color our current experience, but also prime and predetermine our future experience."[13]

As meditation studies continue to gain traction in the West and people gradually begin to experience freedom, a release from the confines of the mind, it is now easier than ever to find a place to start a practice of your own. Just Google "meditation studio" and you'll receive 19 million links!

In a formal setting, Unplug, a Los Angeles-based meditation studio, offers 45-minute drop-in sessions in a serene white space. The studio promotes their offerings in an effort to reach out to people with no meditation experience using the slogan *Hurry Up to Slow Down*. The Path, a roving meditation club that offers weekly sits in New York City, recently launched its first teacher-training program in order to bring mediation to the masses. I predict this is just the first of these kinds of businesses we'll start to see pop up around the United States.

No longer a practice associated with religion, our harried Western culture is craving permission to not do anything and be OK with it. The answer to this might just be meditation.

Reasons to Meditate Now

Best-selling author Peter Bregman has been advising CEOs and senior leaders from major global corporations such as Nike, American Express, and Clear Channel on leadership for years. He advocates for meditation and writes frequently on its benefits for the Harvard Business Review.[1] These are his six reasons to start meditating now:

1. Improve relationships—You will actually be able to fully engage and listen.
2. Increase dependability
3. Enhance performance
4. Make thoughtful decisions
5. Become more clear and intentional in your speech
6. Strengthen your willpower—Not everything will seem so urgent or important.

NOTE

1. Bregman, Peter, "If You're Too Busy to Meditate, Read This," *Harvard Business Review*, October 2012.

MEDITATION DOES OUR BODY GOOD

Over the past 30 years, the effects of meditation have been studied in correlation with addiction, attention, creativity, memory, mental health, physical health, and stress reduction. With a wealth of information out there, it is important to start with an understanding of how meditation affects the neurological pathways in our brain.

If you were to laterally divide the brain, you'd see four surface areas or lobes responsible for different functions. They are:

Frontal Lobe—This area, which contains the medial prefrontal cortex, is known colloquially as the "me center." This area processes information relating to ourselves and to our experiences. It also triggers our body's physical responses. During meditation, this area goes "offline" and we weaken the neural connections, which is actually a good thing. This means we can allow ourselves to have an experience without having an immediate reaction.

Parietal Lobe—Our visual epicenter is located in the parietal lobe, responsible for the processing of sensation and perception and integrating these observations into our brain. Meditation slows the process of sensory information, as your attention is focused on one point, working to shut out outside stimulation.

Occipital Lobe—This is the visual center of our brain. The occipital lobe is responsible for the rapid processing of what our eyes are seeing. This area can remain satiated or even get more active during meditation if you are working on a visualization technique.

Temporal Lobe—Located at the base of the brain is the lobe which processes auditory information. The amygdala, a set of neurons located within the temporal lobe, houses the brain's fear center and responds to emotional stimuli, alerting the brain to problems and activating our fight-or-flight response. During meditation, these neurons are subdued.[14]

For the past decade, the Dalai Lama has encouraged investigation into how the brain responds to meditation. Researchers at the University of Wisconsin-Madison, using Tibetan monks in studies, were able to show a visual representation of how meditation alters the beta waves and their functions of the brain in fMRI scans.[15] It is a fascinating development that has caused a lot of stir in the scientific community, becoming the catalyst for continued research on the effects of meditation on the brain.

The most groundbreaking research to date concerns how meditation alters our brain's gray matter and has come from neuroscientist and meditation practitioner Sara Lazar. In a 2010 study, Lazar's team found that meditation increases the thickness of the prefrontal cortex[16]—the "me center." Why is this important? Our brains start to deteriorate after the first two decades of our lives. It has been suggested that meditation could be the remedy between structural deterioration and functional impairments.[17]

What drew Dr. Lazar into this field of study was personal experience. She started a yoga and meditation practice in graduate school to help cope with the pressure. She found herself

Our Brain on Meditation

The first time I led a meditation visualization exercise on a wellness retreat, we were in a gorgeous outdoor setting in Palm Springs, California; the sun was shining, the air crisp, and the mountains sparkled in the distance. I took inspiration from my surroundings and led attendees on a visual journey up the mountain, asking them to imagine a peaceful room at the top with someone whom they considered a teacher sitting peacefully inside. The meditation was 15 minutes long, and the attendees sat and participated without a sound.

The moment we completed the exercise and opened our eyes, one of the attendees burst into fits of laughter. She shared her visual experience, which had consisted of a litany of characters from ghosts to an old man waiting in the room at the top of the mountain. At some point as she made her way back down the mountain, she burst into flames. As someone new to meditation, she was fully engaged in her experience and it was not until we were finished that she had a physical and emotional reaction.

The entire experience shows how the four lobes of the brain can temporarily recede and disconnect from our actual experiences. The wellness guest was able to have a distinct experience, shutting out outside stimulation, ramping up her occipital lobe with the visualization, and reserving her emotions and judgment until the exercise was complete.

more focused, less stressed, and was so intrigued that as a scientist it changed her perspective. Lazar approached Massachusetts General Hospital, home of Kabat-Zinn's MBSR program, to bring her research here. She found that "participant reported reductions in stress also were correlated with decreased gray matter density in the amygdala, which is known to play an important role in anxiety and stress."[18]

Lazar's conclusions, along with a long-term study out of UCLA, suggest that age-related gray matter atrophy happens less in people who meditate over an extended period of time.[19] As long-term meditators age, their brains get larger and show higher levels of gyrification, or faster information processing.[20] When our brains have more gray matter, we experience more positive emotions and longer lasting emotional stability. Having a regular meditation practice helps protect your brain from age-related tissue decline. Further validation for Lazar's findings came to light in an 8-week MBSR study conducted just last year at Massachusetts General Hospital. Data gathered from the study concluded that there was a direct correlation between reduced stress and decreased gray matter density when novice meditators practiced mindfulness meditation for a minimum of 27 minutes a day.

For people who decide to begin a regular meditation practice, their brains will experience a break down between the neural connections to the "me center." This alteration manifests into positive mental side effects such as decreased anxiety while empathy and rationalization increase. "We know that people who consistently meditate have a singular ability to cultivate positive emotions, retain emotional stability, and engage in mindful behavior,"[21] said Eileen Luders, lead author and a postdoctoral research fellow at the UCLA Laboratory of Neuroimaging. Like Sara Lazar, Luders's research findings showed pronounced structural connectivity of the brain in meditators, which lays the foundation to show that in addition to emotional stability, meditation may slow down aging brain atrophy.

Reshaping the neural pathways of the brain through meditation is also a way to combat daily stress. With only 29% of people doing a good job managing and reducing stress on their own,[22] an attentional-focused practice, such as meditation, can improve the prefrontal cortex's executive function. Reducing stress in this area of the brain allows for better decision-making, problem solving, and helps to resist distraction.

Burnout—the complete physical, mental, and emotional exhaustion caused by chronic stress in the workplace.

As a career consultant who works with CEOs and high-ranking business executives, David Brendel says, "Some problems require more thinking, not less. Sometimes stress is a signal that we need to consider our circumstances through greater self-reflective thought. Mindfulness strategies can prime the mind for sounder rational thinking."[23] By using meditation to reduce our stress, which often manifests itself in the physical forms of anxiety, tension headaches, hair loss, heartburn, IBS, and muscle tension (the list goes on), we can cultivate the tools to avoid burnout, enhance our leadership skills, and steady our minds in the necessary chaos of life.

If you feel like you're suffering from constant fluctuations and chatter of the mind, you are not alone. Researchers at Yale began to examine mindfulness training after discovering that humans have a default network mode that appears to be based in mind wandering; Buddhists have coined this the monkey-mind. The researchers showed correlation between monkey-mind and unhappiness.[24] Using successful mindfulness meditation training, the team was able to show psychological changes such as improved focus, enhanced cognitive flexibility, and reduced reactivity. Additionally, they showed that mindfulness can help prevent relapses into substance abuse or depression, as well as increase the body's ability to tolerate pain. Today, if you have a headache, aspirin may help you cope with the pain, but as a long-term solution, this quick fix is teaching your body to atrophy and limits your ability to deal with distress the next time it arises. mindfulness training, on the other hand, gives us another tool to turn toward to alleviate discomfort.

We all experience stress on some level. Stress wreaks havoc on all parts of our body down to the cellular level. A recent study out of Alberta Canada's Cancer Centre reported that initial mindfulness research shows that physical changes on our telomeres,[25] a part of our DNA which determines how quickly a cell ages, were significantly less degraded when people practiced meditation as a stress reliever. Neuroscientist Clifford Saron came to the same conclusions in his 3-month study[26] for the University of California at Davis, where a mindfulness-based technique was implemented. By working to alleviate stress with mindfulness-based meditation, Dr. Herbert Benson, founding president of the Mind/Body Medical Institute at Harvard Medical School, discovered that physiological changes of relaxation, such as lower heart and respiratory rates, blood pressure, and oxygen consumption, are triggered.

Whether you currently meditate or not, think back to a time or an event that made you feel great—after completing a workout or lounging for a day at the beach, for example. During this happy and relaxed time, the body's dopamine flow increases, improving your mood and possibly releasing a spurt of new ideas. (Entrepreneur Kevin Systrom came up with the idea for Instagram while taking a break from his start-up life in Mexico.) Have you ever had your next brilliant idea come to you in the shower? By performing this rote task, we are able to disengage part of our brain and free it up for divergent thinking, or the ability to generate new ideas or solutions to the same problem.

This concept intrigued researchers at Leiden University in the Netherlands, leading them to explore two forms of meditation and their impact on creativity. Using the aforementioned focused-attention meditation (FA), where participants focus on a particular item or thought, and open-monitoring meditation (OM), where participants notice all aspects of their experience in a nonreactive way, the study explored the specific effects each technique has on creativity. While OM practitioners seemed to experience greater flexibility, fluency, and originality in their thinking, the study concluded that both styles of meditation contributed to an uplifted mood.[27]

I can attest that when I stick to a regular meditation practice, even if it's 5 minutes a day, my overall anxiety and stress level decreases. I am more calm and level-headed in my approach to the day, especially if I'm dealing with a challenging issue at work. But I am thrilled to tell you that positive changes do not stop there. When under mental stress, our brain sends signals to the rest of our body, which affects our physical health. Our endocrine, respiratory, cardiovascular, musculoskeletal, and nervous system can shift and move from a state of quiet to high-alert as a response to what is happening in our brain.[28]

Looking to meditation as a complementary tool, not as a panacea, we can start to decide for ourselves if it could play a role in our overall health. The American Heart Association found that meditation lowers overall risk of heart attacks and strokes.[29] An American Lung Association study concluded that people who learn to meditate were 21% more likely to quit smoking and 25% more likely to abstain from smoking in the following four months than those who tried conventional treatment.[30] And as Jon Kabat-Zinn continues his research, the latest findings show that immune function is boosted in mindfulness meditators.

In 2013, Johns Hopkins completed a study focused on meditation and its effects on depression. The teams findings, published in the *Journal of American Medical Association*, showed that meditation reduced symptoms of depression, anxiety, and pain at the same rate as prescribed antidepressants.[31] In the United Kingdom, researchers have been studying this same correlation for years after Oxford Professor Mark Williams developed Mindfulness-Based Cognitive Therapy (MBCT) as an alternative way to alleviate relapsing into depression without taking medication. The findings have been so successful that the UK National Institute for Clinical Excellence recommends MBCT as the primary treatment for prevention relapse into depression—very forward thinking for a governmental organization!

Some newer studies have been exploring the relationship between mindfulness and chronic pain. Unfortunately, when one is living with chronic pain, suffering is often present, as pain can be debilitating and leave you both mentally and physically exhausted. Dr. Elizabeth Hoge feels that "pain sensations can be mindfully experienced as what they really are, namely sensory experiences."[32] Her 2013 research on pain reveals that with mindfulness training, an experience is possible where, while painful sensations might occur, patients do not necessarily need to suffer from them.[33] This exact experience is what led Mark Bertolini, CEO of one of the United States's largest insurance companies, Aetna, down the path of mindfulness and for doing something unprecedented: introducing mindfulness to over 49,000 of his employees.

MINDFULNESS AT WORK

We have this body of research that shows workplace stress is very bad for health, and we have this other information that says our health costs are way above that of other countries.[34]

—Joel Goh, Harvard Business School

The poor habits that are developed in our teenage years intensify as we move into adulthood. With millennials being the first generation raised on technology, teens (part of Generation Z) are now telling us they feel their stress level during the school year far exceeds what they believe to be healthy, leading them to feel overwhelmed, depressed, or sad as a result. Forty-two percent of teens report they are not doing enough to manage their stress,[35] and whatever coping behaviors they develop now will come with them as they enter the workforce. Is stress the new monkey on their backs? Many business schools think so and are now embracing mindfulness by adding it to MBA coursework.

It is estimated that U.S. businesses lose over $300 billion a year because of stress-related issues, such as absenteeism and health-care complaints, which keep employees from actually working in the office.[36] With rates of stress, burnout, and turnover on the rise, companies from start-ups to Fortune 500s are looking for ways to combat fatigue and apathy and get people back to being excited and engaged.

Author and *New York Times* business reporter David Gelles has been following the mindfulness revolution and the companies who are taking an increased interest in programs to keep current employees mentally fit and attract new ones. Gelles reports the reasons why he believes mindfulness is taking over high-profile companies today[37]:

1. New scientific research shows meditation and mindfulness actually work.
2. Religious connotations and Buddhist roots have been left behind, and people are viewing the practice as secular.
3. With technology and the growing expectation of always being available, we need someone to give us the "OK" to step back and regroup.

Remember our Jolly Good Fellow from Google, Chade-Meng Tan? The *Search Inside Yourself* mindfulness program he developed for Google made them one of the first major companies to recognize that in order to be successful, employees need calm, focused minds when sitting behind a computer for hours each day. Chade-Meng Tan says, "Mindfulness is an idea whose time has come, for a long time practitioners knew, but the science wasn't there. Now the science has caught up."[38]

Mindfulness is sweeping the financial industry, too. While it is more hush-hush, this secret to success is making its way into the hard-partying good old boys clubs and is being used to help turn profits. A May 2014 article in the *London Financial Times* investigated a series of deaths in the financial industry[39] and raised questions about employee stress levels. The piece looked at how people in these high-stress environments were being treated by their higher-ups. While not all companies or employees like to admit it and many declined to be interviewed on the record for the article, people pointed to meditation as the new drug. Not wanting to publicly come across as New Agey, 12% of the people the reporter spoke to admit to participating in mindfulness at work.[40]

Ray Dalio runs the largest hedge fund in the world and is the most vocal advocate for meditation in the financial world. Dalio goes so far as to claim that meditation is the single biggest contributing factor to his success. William George, current Goldman Sachs board member, told the *Financial Times* that "the main business case for meditation is that if you're fully present on the job, you will be more effective as a leader, you will make better decisions and you will work better with other people."[41]

At work, negative stressors come at us from all areas. The perceived actions of customers, clients, bosses, colleagues, and employees, combined with demanding deadlines, are enough to make anyone snap. Turning to the techniques of meditation to elicit the relaxation response allows us to stop analyzing, surrender control, and feel better. Not everyone is ready to step into the limelight and stake a public claim on the effects of meditation. Yet, according to *Bloomberg Business*, financial institutions such as Goldman Sachs Group are embracing meditation, and classes have waiting lists.[42] How practitioners choose to use these tools differ—some aim to make more money, others to sleep better at night, and some as a way to wind down after work.

As a staunch supporter of mindfulness, Arianna Huffington has gone to great lengths to show that you can run a successful business and still take time out of your day to dedicate to your well-being. Huffington writes, "There is nothing touchy-feely about increased profits. This is a tough economy. Stress reduction and mindfulness don't just make us happier and healthier, they're a proven competitive advantage for any business that wants one."[43]

Walter Roth, CEO of Inward Inc, a start-up developed to helping other companies get organized, told the *New York Times* in 2013 that "mindfulness has made me more competitive. Not only do I put fewer things on my to-do list, but I actually get them done and done well. It's like I've learned that to be more successful and accomplish more, I must first slow down."[44]

After a near-death experience resulting from a ski accident, Aetna Health Insurance CEO Mark Bertolini turned to a combination of yoga and meditation as a way to recover and manage his chronic pain. He was skeptical that using these ancient Eastern practices as a form of therapy would have any effect on him—he works for an insurance company, after all, and has access to some of the best doctors in the United States. He was so surprised by his own results that he introduced these programs to his company and, with the backing of Aetna, partnered with Duke University in 2012 to conduct a study of the effects of these wellness programs. This collaboration found that participants gained an additional 69 minutes of productivity each week: 20% reported improvement in their sleep, and 28% felt it helped reduce their overall stress.[45]

Bertolini is thrilled! While the studies prove the effectiveness of this program in the workplace, he is more touched by the results it has given his employees on a personal level. Speaking with *CBS This Morning*[46] in 2015, the CEO relayed instances when people stop him in the hallway to thank him for the programming, as it has helped to save marriages, decrease waistlines, and some have even gone so far as to tell him that these programs have saved their lives. Bertolini is committed to continuing these programs even if you can't boil down the effects into ROI statistics that satisfy shareholders. Bertolini feels he's seen firsthand how investing in his employees is a larger investment in his company.

Soren Gordhamer heard the call and agrees with all the anecdotes. While living in a trailer in northern New Mexico, this divorced, out-of-work, down-on-his-luck guy found the teachings of Eckhart Tolle and Jon Kabat-Zinn and began to apply them to his life. Gordhamer's search for spirituality was merged with this desire to connect with society and work together on larger challenges facing today's world. In 2009, he launched the Wisdom 2.0 conference and invited his social network to an event that merged technology and mindfulness. Now, years later, high-profile CEOs and famous start-up founders make up the conference speakers as well as attendees. Last year's wait-list was over 700 people long.

By breaking down the perceived barriers and turning to science, mindfulness has eschewed its religious roots in the workplace. Instead, companies are recognizing the benefits of a calm, focused mind and its positive effect on creative problem solving. Having a resource such as mindfulness, which increases productivity and helps workers to limit their daily distractions, will only increase profits—something companies can get behind. Marc Lesser, the *Search Inside Yourself* CEO, teaches that "all business is about helping people in some way and you can't do that without focusing on success. The hope is that turning a profit can be done more wisely and compassionately."[47]

General Mills, the U.S.-based food company founded in 1880, has been on the forefront of mindfulness in the workplace and created its own Mindful Leadership Program to reduce stress and increase productivity through meditation and yoga. This program, developed to help employees become better leaders and better individuals, has returned some impressive statistics. The 7-week courses have been beneficial for senior executives as well as mid-level employees. Eighty percent of the executives who have gone through the program report that they now have the tools to make better decisions, while 89% said they have become better listeners.[48] For years, we've known that exercise is good for our bodies. Now we are beginning to understand that mindfulness is exercise for our brain.

While it may seem impossible to start these practices in your office environment, especially if you do not have company support, wellness, and healthy living, guru Deepak Chopra doesn't want to hear excuses. Talking to CNBC's *Squawk Box*, he says, "15 minutes of mindfulness will give you twice as much rest as deep sleep."[49] If you need to work up to 15 minutes, then start with ten. As little as 10 minutes a day, 5 days a week over

How Major Global Corporations Are Embracing Wellness in the Workplace

Aetna Health Insurance—Mindfulness-based wellness programming such as yoga and meditation.

Apple—Meditation rooms as well as expert instructors who lead yoga and myofascial release classes.

Bank of America—Requires employees to take vacation days.

Deutsche Bank—Meditation classes.

eBay—Meditation rooms equipped with pillows and flowers.

Etsy—Offers a digital-free "breathing room" and classes in its Etsy School which teach meditation, juggling, and therapeutic doodling.

General Mills—Meditation and yoga classes through its Mindful Leadership Program.

Google—*Search Inside Yourself* mindfulness programs and lectures.

The Huffington Post—Nap pods and relaxation rooms.

Intel—Created the 9-week Awake@Intel mindfulness program to increase well-being, happiness, and creativity.

L.L. Bean—Asks employees to come up with their own stress-reduction programming, and if a team of 15 committed employees agrees, the company will fund the program.

Nike—Relaxation Rooms for napping.

Rodale Publishing—Built a yoga room at the lobby level showing its significance within the workplace.

Target—Hosts Mindful Leadership retreats and created a Meditating Merchants network in 2010.

Zappos—Full-time life coach on staff.

the course of four weeks can get you on your way to reducing burnout and upping your relaxation.[50]

WHAT DOES SELF-CARE HAVE TO DO WITH IT?

If you consider mindfulness as a means of having a lot of money, then you have not touched its true purpose. It may look like the practice of mindfulness but inside there's no peace, no joy, no happiness produced.[51]

—Thich Nhat Hanh, Zen Master
and mindfulness teacher

Clearly, all of us would benefit from learning how to reduce stress. With no such thing as work/life separation, any tools that we acquire in the workplace will carry into the conversation about reducing the overall stress in our lives. But is learning how to calm your mind the answer alone?

"NO!" is the resounding answer according to many mindfulness advocates. Mindfulness training does have its place at work, as institutionalized programs created for employees can help with relaxation, productivity, and reducing overall healthcare costs. While these are all positive outcomes, New York-based Buddhist psychotherapist Dr. Miles Neale cautions that mindfulness for stress reduction can fail to consider the fact that employees may have to work 12-hour days, be away from their families while traveling, and feel dehumanized by making meaningless products on an assembly line.

So how does one reconcile the stressful demands and expectations of work—of life—without feeling emotionally and spiritually depleted? While we have moved away from the religious roots associated with mindfulness in order to be more accepting of the practice, the concept of self-care was also woven into these ancient teachings and is not something we should dismiss so easily. The World Health Organization defines self-care as "the activities individuals, families, and communities undertake with the intention of enhancing health, preventing disease, limiting illness, and restoring health."[52] Both mindfulness and self-care are constructs that describe how we relate to our experiences and ourselves, whether pleasant or unpleasant, painful or joyful, fearful or fulfilling.

Creating a routine of positive self-care practices can be culturally based and just as crucial to aiding stress reduction. Generations ago, these practices grew out of the lack of health care in
order to be preventative, reactive, and restorative to what ailed
us as a population. Developed throughout the years, self-care
rituals can reflect behaviors according to our cultural habits,
beliefs, practices, and what constitutes our way of life. Somewhere along the way, it was lost in translation, and self-care
became equated with selfishness. We've already proven that
chronic stress leads to burnout, and Gay Becker, of the Institute
of Health and Aging at the University of California, says that
"there is widespread consensus that self-care practices play a
critical role in the management of chronic illness."[53]

What constitutes good self-care? This answer can vary
depending on you as an individual and your needs at various
times throughout your life. The underlying thread should
always be a check and balance to determine whether you are
managing your stress level by creating boundaries, providing
clarity, setting limits, and experiencing feelings of kindness
toward yourself. Yet one thing is clear: self-care has to be a habit.
It is not something that can be done only when you feel like it.
As a matter of fact, the prime time to practice self-care is when
you don't feel like it. Getting enough sleep, providing our bodies
with good nutrition, and fostering meaningful social connections are all examples of self-care, but you cannot turn to these
things as a quick fix; you need to commit to engaging with them
fully in order to reap the benefits long-term.

You're familiar with the saying "happy wife, happy life"?
In our current hurried lifestyle, this expression is just the tip of
the iceberg. We all need to stop waiting around for someone to
give us permission to prioritize ourselves or our happiness. Scientific studies on self-care are currently limited, as there is not one
universal definition. The research available now skews more
toward a spiritual and religious focus, as some of the behaviors
associated with these practices can't be quantified. For example,
many people with illness turn toward religion or spirituality as
comfort, even if up to that point they did not have any lifelong
beliefs.

Spirituality is a complex and multidimensional part of the human experience that is often an individualist path. People can experience spiritual connections via religion or nature or music or art or sporting events—any occurrence that connects you to something else and shows you are not alone. Spirituality has been found to help heal psychiatric disease and heighten emotional intelligence. Practicing the art of hope and forgiveness has been shown to have the strongest negative correlation to anxiety and depressive symptoms,[54] allowing us to feel better, look better, act better, and yes—work better!

All this talk of spirituality makes many doctors and science-minded folks uncomfortable—understandably, as there is no training on this in medical school or in the continuing medical education programming physicians are required to complete every year. This is something that is going to have to change in our society; just because people are uncomfortable with it doesn't mean it should be swept under the rug.

At the Duke University Medical Center in North Carolina, a study of 337 patients who were consecutively admitted to general medicine, cardiology, and neurology services showed that nearly 90% of the patients reported using religion or spirituality to cope with their ailments.[55] Patients found solace in the beliefs and values by which they lived and turned toward the cognitive or philosophic aspects of these beliefs to choose their treatments.

Doctors cannot ignore the experiential and emotional aspects of hope, love, connection, inner peace, comfort, and support, as patients are turning to these areas as part of their whole health care. Today, simply treating a medical diagnosis without considering the person as a whole is no longer acceptable. The rise in preventative care modalities and wellness coping mechanisms has shown this to be true. People are experiencing dramatic changes in all areas of their lives, and stress is the biggest result of these daily pressures. Finding a wellness practice—some combination of mindfulness and self-care, which addresses our whole body—is going to provide support and increase our coping capabilities.

With all our advances in medicine and technology, we are living a decade longer. But with longevity comes pressure to make more of our time on earth and to look good while doing it. Our

Quick and Easy Ways to Incorporate Mindfulness and Self-Care into Your Day

- **Leave for work 10 minutes early**—Upon arrival, sit in your car or on a park bench and do a 5-minute breathing exercise.
- **Take a mid-afternoon coffee break**—But don't actually go for coffee. Instead, do a walking meditation around the block or parking lot. You'll feel refreshed without the side effects of sugar and caffeine.
- **Download a meditation app**—With hundreds of options to choose from, put in a pair of headphones and sneak into the bathroom for a 5-minute break.
- **Turn off your email**—You'll get more done if you designate specific times to checking your email. When working on a big project or something that requires your undivided attention, shut down your email program and reopen it only after you've put some solid hours into the project.
- **Send a calendar reminder**—Our daily routines can be all-consuming. With time slipping away, a little nudge to stop and center isn't a bad thing. Once we get in the habit, it will be easier to cultivate mindfulness in a shorter amount of time, but the key here is consistent practice.
- **Put your phone away**—Stop walking the street or driving in your car while reading your phone. Placing your device into a zipped coat or handbag pocket will alleviate temptation to constantly reach for it.
- **Ask for help**—Knowing how much you can accomplish yourself is a self-care staple. Relying on others doesn't mean you are incapable or not independent, it only means you are human.
- **Get a mentor**—Find someone who can listen and provide sage council.
- **Set boundaries**—Train people to respect your time by powering down your connectivity and decreasing your availability. Saying no or making people wait is not a crime.
- **Make your bedroom a tech-free zone**—Spend your bedroom time relaxing and preparing to sleep. Say goodbye to the TV, computer, and iPad, and find a place for them to live elsewhere in the house.

Western culture is so obsessed with the physical manifestations of aging that the sales of lotions, potions, and Botox continue to soar. Going to the spa and participating in the rituals of self-care are still considered a luxury in the United States and treated as an indulgence. Only now have we begun to understand the role that relaxation plays in stress reduction and our overall health.

The Romans, Russians, and Turks have their baths, which date back centuries. The Swedes and Finns have saunas in their homes, and the Japanese have onsen. Now that the United States is open to understanding the breakthrough medical research on meditation and self-care as stress reduction, we may have just found the key to the fountain of youth: mental antiaging and its low cost is one luxury anyone can afford. After all, sitting pretty is one thing, but having your wits about you will make aging gracefully attainable for everyone.

INTERVIEW: Mindfulness and self-care with Dr. Miles Neale, Buddhist psychotherapist and instructor at the Center for Complementary and Integrative Medicine at Weil Cornell Medical College

The traditional path of mindfulness and meditation is rooted in Buddhist theology and practice; is it possible to become a student of mindfulness without subscribing to a religion?

Dr. Miles Neale: It is certainly possible, and one reason for this possibility is that Buddha is said to have taught 84,000 kinds of teachings, which is one way of saying he was a pragmatist, rather than a dogmatist. The Buddha taught skillfully to the needs and propensities of his students: to some he taught the eradication of vice, to others the cultivation of virtue; to some he taught caring for the self, to others the profound truth of selflessness. Not all these paths offer the same benefits, because clearly something profound is being omitted or deemphasized in each scenario, but they are all legitimate avenues to pursue as long as the meditator is discerning and informed about his or her needs and options.

Mindfulness has gone mainstream and gained support from CEOs and celebrities. They have all turned to meditation for stress reduction and feel it provides a competitive advantage in their business. Are they missing the point or is this how you "sell" meditation to Americans?

DMN: It is a positive step in the right direction that so many people are slowing down, reducing stress, and becoming more attentive through mindfulness meditation. The pace of modern life is spinning out of control, dividing our attention, fragmenting our relationships, and potentially making us sick. However, mainstream mindfulness is not without its issues. Along with all its positive potential, there is a danger in the present trend toward mass-market mindfulness. This danger comes in the form of a capitalistic agenda that procures and codifies mindfulness, selling it as a panacea.

The American public has an appetite for the spectacular and the easy solution. *The Secret*, the yoga boom, and the mindfulness fads are no exceptions. I've coined the term "McMindfulness" to distinguish between the quick-fix, mass-consumption versions of meditation (which do offer some benefits) and the more coherent, long-lasting versions that require commitment and a comprehensive overhaul of one's attitude, lifestyle, and outlook. McMindfulness offers much-needed stress reduction, but fails to address the fundamental mechanisms of interconnectivity and ethical living required for profound human change.

Mindfulness meditation can be used to change your thought process or habitual behavior. One of the most powerful insights I had from an early meditation session was being instructed to bring love and kindness to someone who doesn't like me. How does this rewire the brain and thought patterns? How can one use this technique in a difficult office setting?

DMN: The current neuroscience of brain wiring involves two mechanistic principles: the principle of association and the principle of habituation. When we have an experience, various neurons in our brain fire together and then get wired together, forming a neural network or mental pattern. This is called *association*. During any given experience, a whole range of associations are made between sights, sounds, tastes, smells, tactile experiences, other peoples' facial expressions, how safe we feel, and the meaning, interpretation, or narrative assigned to the event. It's especially true during intense emotional experiences, both positive and traumatic.

If a dog bites you when you're a child, the pain, the dog, and the sense of being unsafe all form an associative neural network. Then, when you're an adult in the park and a dog starts growling, all the associations that wired together fire together, and you feel just as helpless and terrified as you did when you were a child. You fail to make new associations in real time because your past associations color your present perception.

The second related mechanism is the principle of habituation. When we feel intense positive and negative experiences, we tend to respond or react with certain behaviors designed to maintain pleasant or avoid unpleasant sensations in the future. If you do something once, it creates a neural pathway or groove, and if you do the same activity over and over again, the groove gets deeper and more compelling. Through repeated action, these behaviors become automatic, or preconscious, and we no longer need to think of doing them; they are just second-nature or instinctual reactions.

In an office setting, when you see someone with an angry face or tone and you feel threatened or inadequate, you react by accommodating him or her while blaming yourself. You get angry or indignant, and most likely what's happening is that this person is not the actual cause of your distress, but is what I call a "delivery system," eliciting or triggering old associations that are now coloring your experience of the moment. You react largely based on a set of conditioned preconscious responses from countless prior repetitions. We become stuck in a Groundhog Day scenario of unconscious association and compulsive action that further perpetuate future distorted perceptions and experiences of suffering. And that's only half the issue; every time we react this way, we deepen the behavior groove and reinforce the prefab associations, so that we become complicit in our own future negative conditioning.

Seeing through the deceptive veils of our past associations, slowing the movie reel of our minds, and adopting a contemplative lifestyle that reinforces conscious, healthy behavior are all achieved through meditation. By changing your habituated associations and reactions over the long term, you are improving the quality of your inner experience, your relationships at work, and your life.

We live in the age of short attention spans—8 seconds is the average in the United States. Instead of popping pills to overcome ADHD, how can learning a mindfulness technique help you focus?

DMN: Mindfulness, like physical exercise, is an intentional cultivation of awareness or consciousness. There are many forms of this practice. Some techniques cultivate present moment concentration; others cultivate sensitivity to physical reactions. Some cultivate positive emotions such as peacefulness, love, compassion, and even creativity, while other techniques cultivate a realistic outlook and direct insight into the true nature of reality and self. For our distracted, hyper-aroused ADHD culture, training the mind with the narrow-focused, present-centered technique would help balance that distractibility. Every time our mind wanders, we can learn to consciously bring it back again and again, toning and strengthening our mental muscle of concentration.

Ancient texts refer to this as "taming a wild monkey by using a tether" (rope). The tether is a symbol for concentration, securing the beast of distractibility and tethering our attention to one focal point or object like the breath or a sound or an image. If you have a mind, correlated with a brain whose natural capacity is plastic or serviceable, you can train it! And if you want better results, find a personal guide, follow a prescribed program or method, and surround yourself with like-minded individuals for group support.

**Does someone have to sit and meditate for 30 minutes
a day or is doing 5 minutes two times a week better than
not meditating at all?**

DMN: Current research seems to suggest that there is a dose-response or use-dependent association between meditation practice and results. The more you practice, the greater the effect. What seems clear is that consistency is more important than duration, at least initially, in order to rewire the brain based on the principle of habituation. Short practice daily seems to yield better results than long practice once a week. There is also some evidence that 30 minutes of practice twice a day or an hour a day for eight weeks yields positive health outcomes in terms of reduced anxiety and prevention of depressive relapse.

**In 2012, the *Economist* published the article "Think
Yourself Well." Can we use mindfulness meditation
as a technique to make us healthier human beings?
How does this reconcile with traditional medicinal paths?**

DMN: I don't see mindfulness programs replacing high-cost medical interventions, but I do see them extending what's on offer and specifically targeting preventative care. Once you have cancer or several blocked arteries, meditation alone will not likely be enough to reverse these serious medical conditions, although it's not impossible, as we've seen from the work of people like Dean Ornish.

A cultural revolution needs to take place where we wise up and commit to better mental hygiene in order to slow and reverse the so-called pandemic of the diseases of civilization: cancer, heart disease, obesity, depression, diabetes, and addictions. Until that time, I think we'll see surgeries and pharmaceutical and technological interventions for acute and serious medical concerns coexist with so-called soft or holistic or integrative interventions like diet, exercise, meditation, and herbs for preventative and rehabilitative care as well as for chronic ailments.

**It's no surprise that today many people use technology to
engage in mindfulness. While on the outset that may seem**

like a contradiction, it can actually be a positive use of technology and follows the "adapt or die" adage that many businesses thrive on. Do you agree?

DMN: It's amazing that we can preserve, translate, and widely disseminate teachings and practices to anyone with an Internet connection. In my clinical practice, I offer clients 6- to 10-week educational courses that have been archived online where they can access essential theories and practices to support and enhance our individual coaching together. Using an online format undoubtedly saves time and is cost-effective and convenient. But there are some limitations and even drawbacks associated with using technology to teach meditation.

For starters, we live in a time of information overload, and the meditation commodity is no exception. How do people discern what's reliable information from what's not? For beginners, just knowing where to start can be daunting. Marketing and technology go hand-in-hand, so sometimes well-marketed, higher-tech programs have an edge, regardless of the quality of the product.

While technology can make data content available, it will never replace a living, breathing, loving human being. Meditation has been transmitted from teacher to student, mind to mind, for thousands of years, and this subtle, intuitive relationship is an essential variable, an organic vehicle, that is simply irreplaceable in the learning process. Human beings learn and heal best from other human beings in an attended, empathic neural circuitry.

5

GET LOCAL

I spring out of bed in a cold sweat, my pulse racing. Is someone breaking into my apartment? A door cracks open and a shaft of light spills onto the bed. Then I hear a cry: "O perdere così dispiace! Scusa, scusa," as the door abruptly closes again.

Where the hell am I? As things come into focus, I look around the vast room and register the high ceilings, gilded crown molding, and heavy drapes that cascade onto the floor. I run to the window and throw open those drapes.

Italy.

My heart starts to slow as I recognize it now, if only by the cobblestone streets and the taxis whizzing by down below as morning rush hour begins. I scan the street to the left and see the train station, and to the right in the near distance I see the spiked peaks of the Duomo—I'm in Milan.

Have you ever been on a business trip and forgotten what city you are in? Have you ever sat all day in front of your computer and realized at 6pm you have yet to put on pants?

I've done both. Maybe you've done both—at the same time? Today, that was going to end. I was on a business trip in Italy! While I had an afternoon of meetings and an evening event I had to attend, it was time to enjoy my good fortune. I threw on my clothes, stepped out onto the cobblestone street, and made a beeline for a cappuccino. While I stood there drinking it, I made a decision. If I was expected to work 10 hours that day, then the morning would be for me. I needed time to enjoy where I was and rest my brain, my body, and my spirit so that I could show up to work and perform at my best. I spent the next hour wandering the narrow streets and smiling at people I passed in the park. By the time I returned to my hotel room, I was ready to face the long day with a genuine smile on my face.

In today's world, we are so connected to our digital devices we can spend an entire workday "talking" to someone electronically while our tush turns to mush sitting behind a desk instead of interacting with people, places, and situations IRL (in real life). But believe it or not, human interaction with the outdoors, in our communities, and with each other is just as key to whole body well-being as is eating well and exercising often.

My "Get Fit" chapter already took us through the health problems that our sedentary lifestyle causes: shortened life span, heart disease, and type 2 diabetes among others, so we know we should be moving more on a daily basis. We've also established that sitting is the new smoking, and being indoors is associated with more sitting. In this chapter, we'll explore how getting outdoors and coming face-to-face your tribe helps prevent or stave off these ailments and others. When we get up from behind our desk or leave our hotel room or take time to smile at those we pass on the street, we're connecting to people, places, and yes, real life around us.

IT'S A CONCRETE JUNGLE OUT THERE

"Just get out of the car." I can't tell you how many times I heard my father, a horticulturist, say this. With his hand on the open backdoor, he would lean down looking at my brother and me as we sulked in the backseat of the car having just pulled up to another park. It was a Saturday or a Sunday or a family vacation, and it always seemed to involve nature and history. And we hated it! Or so we pretended, until some twenty minutes later when we were scurrying over rocks or marveling at a massive form of nature or racing each other through the woods. Growing up in the suburban Midwest, I may have been a part of the last generation to play outside all day without checking in at home.

We'd grab our bikes and ride around the neighborhood or head down to the local park to hang out with our friends for hours on end, doing nothing but trying to catch crawfish in the stream or goofing around on the swings at the playground. (Nowadays, my nephew is proficient with an iPad at age three.)

Before it was used as a euphemism for going to the bathroom, going out for your morning constitutional meant a walk. This phrase was derived from the word constitution.

Constitution—a person's physical state with regards to vitality, health, and strength.

As our daily lives grew busier and we were expected to be in the office earlier and earlier, the morning constitutional fell by the wayside, which is unfortunate for both our minds and bodies. Our indoor environments are ripe with pollutants (cleaning products, air fresheners, dust, mold, animal dander) which expose us to poorer air quality than if we were outdoors.[1] Whenever possible, we should be throwing our windows open to circulate the air to improve the quality, or better yet, throwing on our coats and getting outside to inhale a deep fresh breath.

Today, living in a concrete jungle, I don't miss suburban life, but I do crave nature and relish the times I am able to leave the city for wide-open spaces. Daily life, especially in an urban setting or in a high-powered job, is depleting. You are constantly bombarded with stimuli and give of your emotions and personal space, while at the same time expending tremendous amounts of energy protecting yourself physically (walking down the streets with our shoulders hunched inward), mentally (assessing every person walking toward you for signs of danger), and emotionally (seeking therapy or reprieve of some kind). In this setting, the body's fight-or-flight response is constantly in fight mode, leading to a continuous hum of chronic stress which manifests as full-body pain and distress.

Doctors and coauthors Randloph Nesse and George Williams explain this in their book *Why We Get Sick*: "Natural selection has not had time to revise our bodies for coping with fatty diets, automobiles, artificial light, and central heating. This mismatch between our design and today's environment may account for many preventable modern diseases."² Historically, societies, including our forefathers, used nature and its resources for the healing properties it provides. Many of our modern pharmaceutical treatments, such as artemisinin used to treat malaria³ and lovastatin used to lower cholesterol,⁴ have been derived from phenomena that originated in a natural setting. Doctors used to prescribe "fresh air" as a curative, and today, functional medicine doctors such as Frank Lipman, Alejandro Junger, and Andrew Weil all advocate for healing through food that is grown in nature. Yet we've moved so far away from our direct relationship to the earth in such a short time that our bodies have not had time to adapt. With so little free time on our hands, how do we get back to nature?

Those times I get to drive over the bridge and head out of the city for a hike or get on a plane for a remote part of the world fill me back up and return me to a calm, focused, more productive, less stressed state. It turns out there is science to explain this physiological reaction: attention restoration theory (ART). ART was developed in the 1980s by psychology professors Rachel and Stephen Kaplan. The theory states that spending time in nature, an environment that does not want anything from us, allows us to use our indirect attention, which requires no effort on our part at all.⁵

William James, psychologist, doctor, and philosopher, explained in the early 1900s that our attention could be classified into two categories: direct (voluntary) and indirect (involuntary). Our direct attention requires focus and allows us to read a book, pay attention in meetings, and avoid being hit by a car when crossing the street. After a while, this intense focus becomes fatiguing to our body and mind. Indirect attention is involuntary and happens when our minds wander, when we daydream or stare at the clouds going by out the window. Nature, according to the principles of ART, helps facilitate our indirect attention and restores our ability to successfully use our direct attention.

Our environment plays a critical role in how we think and how we behave. Current research shows that the average American spends 93% of their entire life inside: 87% enclosed in buildings and 6% in a vehicle.⁶ With a whole wide world out there to explore, this is a shocking statistic. In his 2005 book *Last*

Child in the Woods, author Richard Louv (whom I interviewed for this chapter) defined this epic problem as nature deficit disorder.

Nature deficit disorder—the human cost of alienation from nature, among them: diminished use of senses, attention difficulties, and higher rates of physical and emotional illnesses.[7]

Louv goes on to state that nature deficit disorder (NDD) "can be detected in individuals, families, and communities. NDD can even change human behavior in cities, since long-standing studies show a relationship between the absence or inaccessibility of parks and open space with high crime rates, depression, and other urban maladies."[8] With nature being bulldozed to build housing and the rainforests being raided to make needed building materials, it's no surprise that our natural environments are shrinking in favor of urban settings.

Since the 1980s, there has been a 20% decline in visits to U.S. national parks[9] and a shift away from nature-based recreation in favor of indoor activity: think video games, which paved the way for the Internet, which accounts for our indoor screen time, leaving no time to head outdoors into nature. In 2008, the world reached a huge milestone, which shifted the balance of the planet: there are now more people living in urban areas than outside of them.[10] That same year, a study found that children living with attention deficit hyperactivity disorder (ADHD) scored higher on tests of concentration after a walk through a park instead of a walk through a residential neighborhood.[11] At the moment, there is no direct connection between these statistics, but the information should give us pause.

The millennial generation was the first to be raised on technology. Looking at this demographic, 80% of kindergarten-aged kids were computer users, and by the time they reached 18 they were spending an average of seven and a half hours every day in front of a screen.[12] Figuring in the total waking hours of this group and how they spent their time means that an average of 15 to 25 minutes a day were spent outdoors playing or participating in sports.[13] In these formative years, cognition and attention are not fully developed, so even without a screen coming into

Get More Nature Now

- Open two windows for 10 minutes so that a cross-breeze can clear out the stale air and lingering pollutants.
- Kick off your shoes and walk barefoot on the grass to calm your nervous system.
- Move your desk in front of a window. If this is not possible, then a few times a day walk to a window and gaze out for a moment.
- Move your meetings outdoors. If you can't convince your coworkers to join you for a walking meeting, then set up a table and chairs in the sun.
- Take a different route home through the countryside. Stop to get out of the car and take 5 deep, present-centering breaths before continuing.

play, children have less attentional control (what they choose to pay attention to) than adults and are often easily distracted.

Jane Clark, professor of kinesiology and dean of the School of Public Health at the University of Maryland, has referred to today's child-rearing approach as the age of "containerized kids."[14] As adults have evolved to take on a sedentary lifestyle, we have passed our way of relating to the world down to our children. We make infants and toddlers sit in car seats, high chairs, and bouncers, and starting at age five, in some cases earlier, kids are expected to sit in a chair at school and stay still while they listen to a teacher. Oftentimes, after-school schedules are packed with language classes, music lessons, or extra tutoring. With recess and Physical Education being cut across the country, when are kids supposed to find time to run around outside and engage in creative play? When are they going to find time to just be kids?

As adults, we need to move to counteract the effects of being sedentary. Combining exercise and nature packs a one-two punch for both our physical health and mental state. In 2005, the *International Journal of Environmental Health Research* released a study that looked at the outcomes of outdoor exercise. The findings showed that exercise in both pleasant rural and urban settings had more positive effects on self-esteem than exercising indoors.[15] Newer research out of Stanford University looked specifically at walking indoors on a treadmill facing a blank wall versus outdoors and its impact on creativity. While both settings improved the free flow of ideas, getting outdoors elicited the most novel and highest quality responses.[16]

This is great news for the office. On days when you're brainstorming or are up against a particularly challenging issue and you feel like you've hit a wall, a walk outside will get your creative juices flowing. According to University of Essex researcher Jules Pretty, "You get a very substantial benefit from the first five minutes. We should be encouraging people in busy and stressed environments to get outside regularly, even for short bits of time."[17]

When we spend time in nature, the body expends less energy filtering out the things we don't need. With more physical space between you and another person, you don't constantly have to evaluate other people's energy coming your way. The body can slowly start to relax, which allows blood pressure, cholesterol, and stress levels to drop.[18] Consistent contact with nature also allows for the regulation of the adrenal and nervous systems,[19] both of which are long-term preventative health measures that will help you lead a longer, more healthful life. It's never too late to start spending time in nature. Even if you commit to the outdoors starting at 70 years of age, by the time you reach 77, you'll have less musculoskeletal pain, fewer sleep issues, less logistic regression, and better overall health than a 77-year-old who has not regularly taken advantage of the outdoors in the previous seven years.[20]

But don't wait until you retire to make it outdoors. Currently, most adults, even healthy ones, are lacking in vitamin D, often referred to as the sunshine vitamin. Vitamin D helps your body absorb calcium, which is needed for healthy bones and teeth. So even if you get enough calcium in your diet, if you don't have enough vitamin D in your system, that calcium isn't able to work for you. Some studies have even suggested that those lacking in vitamin D can have future health issues such as osteoporosis, cancer, and depression.[21] So it's important to make it a point to get outdoors a few times a week and soak up some vitamin D. Take that walk around the block at lunch. Sit on a

Get Grounded

When I first started exploring the concept of grounding or earthing, the reaction I would get from my clients was a look akin to "oh, that hippy shit." I get it: running around barefoot on the grass is literally thought of as child's play or conjures up images of longhaired women skipping through a field of flowers. In 2012, the *Journal of Environmental and Public Health* published an article diving deep into current research, which suggests that our disconnection from the earth may be a major contributing factor to our physiological dysfunction. Pulling information from 7021 studies, the article authors found emerging evidence that being barefoot outdoors, grounding us into a connection with the Earth, may be effective at reducing chronic stress, inflammation, pain, and poor sleep.[1] While much more research is needed in the field, we can all agree that getting outside and sticking our feet in the grass or digging our toes in the sand while on vacation produces a smile, and sometimes that sense of enjoyment is all you need to overcome a case of the Mondays.

NOTE

1. Chevalier, Gaetan, et al., "Earthing: Health Implications of Reconnecting the Human Body to the Earth's Surface Electrons," *Journal of Environmental and Public Health* (2012), article ID 291541, http://dx.doi.org/10.1155/2012/291541

bench in the sun while you sip your morning coffee. Skip the hotel treadmill in the morning and instead run outdoors in the surrounding neighborhood.

Nature can also heal us without direct contact. In 1972, healthcare researcher Roger Ulrich began a hospital study on U.S. patients recovering from gallbladder surgery by dividing recovery patients into two groups: those with a tree view out their hospital window and those with a brick building view. At the end of this nine-year study, the collected data revealed that those patients who enjoyed a nature view needed less pain-relieving medication, were more cooperative with the hospital staff, and on average went home a day sooner than those who spent their recovery time staring at the building view.[22] Imagine yourself in this situation. Most of us would prefer to reap the benefits of a nature view, too. In addition to the scientific outcomes, empirical evidence indicates that knowing that nature is available and having the ability to experience it, even through a window, will generally make us happier, healthier people.[23]

HUG A TREE

> It is not so much for its beauty that the forest makes a claim upon men's hearts, as for that subtle something, that quality of air, that emanation from old trees, that so wonderfully changes and renews a weary spirit.[24]
>
> —Robert Louis Stevenson

In 1982, a curious thing happened in Tokyo. A man by the name of Tomohide Akiyama proclaimed that the country was in need of healing in the form of nature, specifically the act of shinrin-yoku, or forest bathing. Akiyama, minister of Agriculture, Forestry, and Fisheries at that time, claimed that shinrin-yoku could be used to improve mental and physical health regardless of age or background.[25] In order to properly engage in shinrin-yoku, one had to set aside a few hours and head into the forest with no distraction, using the body's five senses to engage with the surroundings.

As the Japanese began to take to the forests, scientists at Nippon Medical School in Tokyo started to study shinrin-yoku's effects and they made some amazing discoveries: participating in this wellness activity proved to have positive effects on both physical and mental health. First was a look into how cerebral activity differed from an urban setting to a forest environment. The study found that shinrin-yoku was effective, relaxing the body and brain activity of those who lived in urban surroundings.[26] Further research found that engaging in 2 to 4 hours of forest bathing on two consecutive days allows for the inhalation of phytoncides, antimicrobial compounds emitted by trees and plants. Breathing in these compounds showed an increase of 40% in white blood cell activity, the body's natural defense system, and anticancer proteins, and a follow-up a month later revealed the body retained a 15% increase in these cells.[27]

In Korea, a forest bathing experiment was undertaken to study shinrin-yoku's healing effect on severe depression. Researchers engaging patients in psychotherapy sessions outdoors found reduced cortisol (stress) levels, improved heart rate variability (interval between heart beats), and reduced overall depressive symptoms, leading to a remission rate of 61% higher in the forest bathing group than the group that just used medication alone.[28] All of this data on adults was becoming quite compelling, so the scientific focus started to shift to the younger generation and the behavioral impact nature could have started at a young age.

In 2011, the Centers for Disease Control estimated that 6.4 million American children under the age of 17 had been professionally diagnosed with attention deficit hyperactivity disorder (ADHD), and the number continues to rise.[29] Several studies have suggested that allowing kids to spend time in nature reduces attention deficit symptoms even if a child has not responded to medication. Researchers who looked at the effects of nature and ADHD medication found that some children were able to cut their dosage in half just by spending some time communing with the outdoors.[30]

Even if you do not suffer from ADHD, many of us have attention fatigue, a temporary condition, where at the end of a long day we feel we can no longer pay attention. The cure for attention fatigue is ART, allowing us the opportunity to rest both our cognitive and nervous systems. Richard Louv, along with other researchers in the field, feels that nature deficit disorder and attention fatigue, possibly even ADHD, "can be recognized and reversed, individually and culturally,"[31] by adding quality time in nature back into a wellness routine.

After three decades of research, the Japanese government officially recognized shinrin-yoku as a healthful practice and designated certain areas of it (67% of forestland) as forest therapy bases and roads. Forest bathing made a big splash in the United States in 2015 when the Global Wellness Institute named it a top wellness therapy to watch. Many U.S.-based programs

Tips to Get the Most out of Your Forest Bathing Experience

- Plan the time and terrain you are going to cover on your journey so you don't get tired. Remember, this is supposed to be reinvigorating.
- Find a place along the way where you can sit and rest. Take a deep breath and soak in everything around you.
- If the goal is to boost your body's immunity, or natural killer cell activity (a type of white blood cell)s, you need to do an overnight. Find a campsite or bed and breakfast (B&B) surrounded by nature and head out over the weekend to explore.
- If you don't have time to get out into a national park or forest, a few hours in a dense city park can significantly reduce anxiety and depression. Try places like New York City's Central Park, a hiking trail such as Escondido Canyon in Malibu, California, or your local botanical garden.

are popping up in places like Northern California and the Pacific Northwest, so joining a regular group for some quality time in nature is becoming a no-brainer.

FRESH AIR FOR THE SOUL

> *When they go fishing, it is not really fish they are after.*[32]
>
> —E. T. Brown

When Professor J. Arthur Thomson addressed the British Medical Association in 1914, he put forth the notion that our minds were being diseased by the constant rush and racket of developing civilization and that nature held the key to good mental health.[33] Over a hundred years later, I totally agree with the guy. Even if you don't live in a major city, the modern life happening around us right now is a constant stimulant. People who cannot access nature outside their front door have turned to meditation or medication to try and cultivate some of the calm that nature can provide.

Combat SAD

Seasonal affective disorder (SAD) is a type of depression that is tied to the seasonal changes of the environment. If SAD affects you, you will typically start to see signs such as fatigue, low energy, depression, and moodiness appear in the fall months and continue throughout winter. This seasonal disorder happens when you are exposed to reduced levels of sunlight, which causes serotonin (the mood-balancing hormone) levels to drop. It can also affect how the body produces melatonin—leading to changes in sleep patterns. Symptoms shift again and will disappear as warmer weather returns and daylight hours increase.

If you are affected with SAD, try to combat it by:

- **Getting Outside**—Anytime that you can expose your body to direct sunlight will be beneficial, especially if you can do so first thing in the morning.
- **Bring the Outdoors In**—Throw open the blinds, add a sky light to your home, buy some plants for your desk, and make sure you have nothing obstructing your view of the outdoors if you work by a window.
- **Wake Up Naturally**—Some people switch to a dawn simulator alarm clock, which will fill your room with gradually increasing light no matter what is happening outdoors, allowing you to sync your circadian rhythm to the times of year you feel happiest.
- **Take a Vacation**—Getting away somewhere warm and sunny in the winter will do wonders for your entire well-being, plus it will break up your winter into more manageable chunks of time.

Like meditation and medication, time in nature can decrease anxiety and negative moods. Being surrounded by nature can produce powerful rehabilitation results—it's no accident that at the turn of the nineteenth century, the country's health resorts and sanitariums were set in the woods on acres of natural expanse. Over 35 years ago in the *Journal of Leisure Research*, it was reported that spending time in a park within a city reduced anxiety and lowered levels of sadness.[34] This is because going from the busy city streets into an urban green space has immediate, real-time effects such as drops in frustration and hyperactivity and an increase in calm.[35]

A park, even if buildings surround it, triggers our parasympathetic (rest and digest) nervous system, as relaxation allows for the stress to start melting away.

For those who suffer from depression, walks in nature have been shown to significantly reduce depressive feelings and the negative effects that come with being depressed. Studies in both the Netherlands[36] and the United Kingdom[37] have shown that people who live near a park experience less depressive episodes and anxiety. If you can find a friend to walk with you, that's even better, as having a buddy who is relying on you for their time in nature will hold you more accountable. Having this direct contact with the area in which you live or work creates a bond, a sense of stewardship for the environment in which you interact. Spending time in nature reminds you just how awesome and awesomely big the world is. Even if you do not have a medical diagnosis, time in nature has been shown to reduce overall stress hormones, decrease blood pressure, calm the parasympathetic nervous system,[38] and improve positive emotions.

After reviewing various studies performed within their borders, the UK Department of Health was able to establish a direct link between human connection to a natural environment and its influence on overall well-being. Now the government lists the use of nature as a determinant of public health, stating that improving citizen's access and involvement in nature could reduce government spending by as much as $3 billion dollars.[39] Even if you can't get outside at regular intervals, adding some plants to your home or workspace will improve your mood and your productivity.[40]

REACH OUT AND TOUCH SOMEONE

> *I want to be around people who dream and support and do things.*[41]
>
> —Amy Poehler

The idea of getting local isn't just about spending time in nature. We live in a society that has evolved from communal living—needing each other to survive, to help us eat, to help raise our children—to now having smaller nuclear connections and using the Internet as a barrier from real human interaction. As humans, we are a social species that need real, meaningful connections to grow, flourish, and increase our social wellness.

Loneliness is a real epidemic in our society today. In 2006, researchers from Duke University published a study in the *American Sociological Review* that noted that over the course of their twenty-year study, the drop among close confidants of their subjects decreased by 30%.[42] While there is some debate about applying the study's finding to generalized social isolation in America, the study sheds light on how social connection is drastically changing as our society evolves and technology takes on an even bigger role.

Physical isolation is different from loneliness. When someone is alone, it is because they do not have anyone to rely on, to share their intimate moments with, or to turn to in times of trauma. You're probably familiar with the concept of being surrounded by hundreds of people but still feeling lonely. Loneliness heightens sensitivity to social threats and can impair brain function and sleep, as well as mental and physical well-being.[43] Dr. Matthew Lieberman writes in his book *Social: Why Our Brains Are Wired to Connect* that our brains are made to reach out and interact with others, and that from a young age our brains learn to experience social pain, and therefore, we spend time trying to find ways to avoid it.

When we are not part of a group or community, our physical health is drastically affected. Research shows that if a person is alone for a prolonged period of time, the risk of early death increases by 14%.[44] When someone experiences sustained loneliness, the body focuses on staying healthy in the moment, fighting immediate threats such as colds and flus, not long-term ones.[45] This leaves a person exposed to long-term diseases like cancer and heart failure due to a weakened immune system as well as the chance of developing dementia, which increases by 64%[46] when loneliness is persistent.

Find Your Tribe

Not sure how to stay connected to your community or don't know where to start if you've moved to a new place? See if any of these ideas spark an interest for you:

- **Reach out to coworkers**—Whether you approach it as networking, a chance to connect with a coworker, or just time with a person you have some common ground with, you know you'll at least have something to talk about.
- **Join a religious organization or community center**—Oftentimes you hear of empty-nesters finding religion again. While for some the religion itself may play a role, for others it's just about finding a community of like-minded people with which to spend time. If religion is not your thing, head to your local community center and join a group activity (forest bathing group, anyone?) that appeals to you.
- **Volunteer**—Helping someone other than yourself makes you feel good. Those positive emotions increase self-esteem and will make it easier to form meaningful connections.
- **Accept invitations**—Even if there are a million reasons to say "no," the more you say "yes" when people invite you out, the more invitations you'll receive. If you're on the fence, give yourself a time limit of 30 minutes, and if you're not having a good time, then leave.
- **Play Pokémon Go**—This new augmented reality game is sweeping the globe, and while it definitely leads you around the world via your screen, you have the opportunity to make real-world connections at each stop. Be it exploring landmarked areas, spending time in parks, or striking up a conversation with someone you already have something in common with, it could be the new way to get off the couch and enjoy the world around you.

Faced with such uncertainty in the world, it's natural to look for a group of like-minded people that will make you feel grounded and connected to something tangible. Having a connection to a tribe can alleviate unhappiness, increase your sense of security, and increase your overall view of life satisfaction. Weak social ties to a community have been shown to be just as harmful to one's health as smoking a pack a day.[47] When you are able to surround yourself with healthy relationships, it encourages healthy habits. A healthy relationship, as defined by John Cacioppo, director of the University of Chicago's Cognitive and Social Neuroscience Department, is a connection with someone who provides positive affirmations, face-to-face, mutually rewarding contact, and connection beyond your individual existence.[48] Having these meaningful connections not only helps to validate your being, but also allows you to be responsible and have more pride of "ownership" over your body, as you want to present your best self. When you have people in your life to care about or that care about you, such as children or a new love, better hygiene and more risk adverse behavior becomes your natural choice.

Our need for connection starts as babies. Decades ago, the infant mortality rate was linked to human contact or a lack of it. When the medical community began to analyze the data in the 1940s, they were stunned to learn that infants without social interaction or a human connection would die before they reach seven months.[49] This discovery forced policy changes in the country's orphanages and created a shift in the way healthcare in hospitals was provided, and touch therapy became crucial to their survival. If you've ever received a massage or gotten a bear hug from someone whom you care about, then you understand the feeling and effects of nonsexual physical contact. In these moments, you can feel your heart rate slow, your stress levels drop, and any anxiety or depression ebbing—this is your body's relaxation response, and it's in these moments that we restore our body to homeostasis.

The same holds true as we age. We've all heard stories of couples that have been married for decades dying within hours of each other, or people who retire in their 80s only to pass away shortly thereafter. The older we get, the more inclined we are

Five Reasons to Call Your BFF Right Now

- Boost your happiness level
- Reduce stress
- Give you a sense of purpose
- Provide emotional support
- Let you be your true self

to stay home and not venture out alone. Even if we had robust social connections earlier in life, if we do not actively engage in keeping up the connections, we can enter a period of social isolation. As relationships wane and social isolation sets in, you are 4.2 times more likely to develop an illness than people who maintain diverse social connections.[50] These deep social connections are a central source of emotional support and overall well-being for many people.

A look at the state of our social connections over the last 50 years appeared in a 2013 article in *The Atlantic.* Author Emily Smith noted that as society becomes more prosperous, we become more individualistic, more isolated. "We volunteer less. We entertain guests at our homes less. We are getting married less. We are having fewer children. Over the same period of time that social isolation has increased, our levels of happiness have gone down, while rates of suicide and depression have multiplied."[51]

Finding a community you fit into and can relate to, one that offers you support in hard times is crucial to your well-being. With social media and screen time taking over our waking hours, it's never been more important to connect with both a real-life community and the outdoors. The University of Michigan released a study in 2013 that showed the more young adults used Facebook over a 2-week period, the more their life satisfaction declined.[52] When you are able to find your tribe offline, you are more likely to become a contributing member as being around like-minded people increases your self-esteem and gives you a touch point to care about. This holds true for both the environment and the people that surround you. Integrating nature and community into your life, even if it's for short spurts throughout the day, leads to better physical, mental, and emotional health as well as less social isolation and violence.[53] People of all ages benefit from getting local and making connections, since it's never too late to start, put this book down right now and call your bestie to say hello.

INTERVIEW: How connecting with nature and community can help heal us with Richard Louv, chairman emeritus of the Children & Nature Network and author of nine books including *Last Child in the Woods: Saving Our Children from Nature-Deficit Disorder*

In your 2005 book *Last Child in the Woods*, you coined the phrase "nature deficit disorder"—our alienation of nature, diminished use of senses, attention difficulties, and higher rates of physical and emotional illnesses. Ten years later, has our collective nature deficit disorder worsened?

Richard Louv: The barriers between people and nature remain challenging, but we're seeing some change. In the United States, we're beginning to see progress among state legislatures, schools and businesses, civic organizations, and government agencies. Family nature clubs (multiple families that agree to show up for a hike on Saturday) are proliferating. In September 2012, the World Congress of the International Union for the Conservation of Nature (IUCN) cited "adverse consequences for both healthy child development ('nature-deficit disorder') as well as responsible stewardship for nature and the environment in the future," and then passed a resolution titled "The Child's Right to Connect with Nature and to a Healthy Environment." This connection is, indeed, a human right. And the acknowledgment of that is progress. In September 2015, the new White House initiative called "Every Kid in a Park" went into effect, where all 4th-grade students and their families will have free admission to national parks and other federal lands and waters. While we're seeing progress, many barriers between children and nature still exist, and some are growing. We need leadership at every level—

policy makers, parents, grandparents, healthcare professionals, teachers, business people—and in every country to bring down barriers such as urbanization without nature and value how nature enriches our society.

A study published in the *Archives of Pediatrics & Adolescent Medicine*[54] showed that children have trouble concentrating in school before 8:30am. One suggestion that's been offered to address this is to hold Physical Education at the start of every day, giving kids time outdoors and allowing them to "wake up." In addition to providing kids with nature, might this affect the growing number of depression and ADHD diagnoses in children today?

RL: Even without the research, that makes practical sense. The research on nature's impact on education and health has greatly expanded over the last few years. Because researchers have turned to this topic relatively recently, most of the evidence is correlative, not causal—but it tends to point in one direction: experiences in the natural world appear to offer great benefits to psychological and physical health and the ability to learn for children and adults. The research strongly suggests that time in nature can help many children reduce the symptoms of attention deficit hyperactivity disorder and can be powerful therapy for such maladies as mental depression.

Certainly, Physical Education is a wonderful way to start the day. Many physicians recommend exercise as part of a health-promoting program, and outdoor play of any sort is good, but we do need a wider array of approaches—including a greater focus on nature experience. The emerging information on green exercise—free play in a natural green space—suggests that this particular kind of outdoor activity may have added antioxidant properties. The calming, mood-enhancing benefits of green exercise are often cited, as are green exercisers' improvements in self-esteem, concentration, and test scores. Researchers at the University of Essex in England have been looking into the benefits of green exercise for a number of years and have documented improvements in psychological well-being through nature-based exercise.

Pope Francis' 2015 encyclical called for a drastic universal change in our lifestyle in order to more mindfully care for our planet. The Pope linked our environmental issues to our social ones, calling into question corporate responsibly for our well-being. What kind of benefits could a company reap by investing in its employees' well-being?

RL: Incorporating nature into time at work is smart from a business and economics standpoint. There are a number of studies and real-life examples demonstrating that incorporating nature into business and the workplace can produce new products, and for employees, potential reductions in lost work time, absenteeism, and turnover rate. Outdoor time is ideal for improving well-being, but even infusing the design and everyday experience of our workplaces can make us *more* productive. Research suggests that direct and indirect contact with nature can help with recovery from mental fatigue and the restoration of attention, as well as help restore the brain's ability to think. Having green plants in your cubicle can make a big difference in your psychological well-being. Even images of nature—photos, paintings, videos—have been shown to have a calming effect on people, but the real thing is really what works best.

Former New York City mayor Michael Bloomberg created a lot of public policies aimed at improving the wellness of the city's residents during his 12-year tenure. One of his legacies was adding green space back into the urban landscape. Does an initiative like this help a fast-paced capital-minded city function better as a whole?

RL: Definitely. A healthier habitat increases human-nature social capital for everyone's benefit. There is an enormous impact to creating parks, open space, and nearby nature in cities including more social bonding, a positive economic impact on public mental and physical health, education, and jobs. Measures of the influence of the natural world on child and adult obesity and depression, for example, could be translated into direct and indirect costs of health care and lost productivity. The positive impact on property values could also be measured and reported. A green city can also reshape health care, tourism, and law enforcement in positive ways. If we are going to have meaningful experiences with nature, we are going to have to rethink nature within cities.

A growing number of planners and educators are working toward increasing the natural or naturalistic play spaces available to urban children, and many civic leaders are now aware of the nature deficit problem. Family nature clubs, a grassroots movement uniting families and helping parents and kids reduce their anxiety about venturing into the outdoors, are popping up all over. To connect to that nature, we can walk in our neighborhoods, get to know these pockets of nature, find out how to protect them, and then learn new ways to bring *more* nature to the urban areas. At least one study has shown that urban parks with the highest levels of biodiversity happen to be the parks with the greatest psychological benefits for human beings. Cities can, in fact, become engines of biodiversity. Groups that help people really see where they live, that foster a sense of place, are growing in size and number. As the poet and farmer Wendell Berry says, "You can't know who you are until you know where you are."

Nippon Medical School in Tokyo conducts experiments to test the effects of shinrin-yoku, or forest bathing: spending leisurely time in nature and the effects it has on our physical, emotional and mental well-being. Currently, a big trend in the wellness sector, could forest bathing be the answer to curing nature deficit disorder?

RL: One of the tenets of the nature principle is that the more high-tech our lives become, the more nature we need. Digital technology is, of course, not going away, so we need nature in our lives as a balancing agent, now and in the future, more than ever. In fact, we need what I've called the Hybrid Mind: knowing both the virtual and the natural world. The ultimate multitasking is to live simultaneously in both the digital and the physical world, using computers to maximize our powers to process intellectual data and natural environments to ignite all of our senses and accelerate our ability to learn and to feel; in this way, we would combine the resurfaced "primitive" powers of our ancestors with the digital speed of our teenagers.

You've said you'd rather be fishing than writing. What are some simple ways busy people can add more nature into their lives right now?

RL: Schedule outdoor time. Direct experiences in nature: make getting outside in a natural area an intentional act—a healthful habit, if you will—so that it becomes part of your life. It can be as simple as planning regular walks around a local park, taking picnics, or learning how to garden in containers on the back stoop. You can encourage wildlife rehabilitation or go canoeing, birding, fishing, or camping. You can join or start a family nature club. My new book, called *Vitamin N*, includes 500 actions that people can take to enrich the health and happiness of their families and communities—and to help create a future that we'll all want to go to.

6

GET FOOD

Growing up in the Midwest, my diet wasn't exactly meat and potatoes—more like meat and salad—but heavy on the carbs nonetheless. I learned some good habits (vegetables at every dinner) and some bad (leftover dessert for breakfast), which have stuck with me or gone by the wayside throughout the years. Summertime in the late 1980s had us stopping roadside to buy sweet corn direct from the farmers or heading out to pick our strawberries on the weekends. We would sit down to home-cooked family meals at 5pm nearly every night. And starting at 14, my brother and I were each given the responsibility of creating and cooking one of those meals each week.

Our weekly staples became chicken parmesan, ground beef lasagna, chicken and vegetable stir-fry, and flank steak on the grill, all served with an iceberg lettuce salad. When my father traveled for work, my mom took a break from cooking, and we were treated to McDonald's or Wendy's and shared a pint of Ben and Jerry's after dinner. When I was sixteen, I stopped eating red meat (must have been a trend), but essentially I became a junk food vegetarian, surviving on pasta, pizza, cheese, and crackers along with my nightly salad and chicken as my protein. Our big extended family holiday dinners were full of buffets of food, but oftentimes these main courses were just place holders until the desserts came out: cookies, brownies, mocha tort, and cake, followed by morning brunches of delicious sugary coffee cake.

In the summer, if we'd vacation with our cousins at the beach, the house was always full of M&Ms, and every night we'd go out for ice cream. In high school, after my team would win a volleyball game, we'd celebrate with pizza and talk of carbo-loading before our next big match. Fat-free snacks were wildly popular at the time, and during school lunches, kids would break out the Snackwells or stand in line to get fat-free frozen yogurt.

When I left home for college, I actually lost weight. I never packed on the "Freshman 15," even though every Friday and Saturday night of that year was spent in the corner deli ordering breaded chicken sandwiches with lots of mayonnaise. Living in New York City opened my eyes to a world of food that was fresh, flavorful, varied, and at my fingertips. Sushi, Korean barbeque, Spanish tapas, Indian, Vietnamese, Thai, mixed green salads, endives, hearts of palm, avocado that wasn't in the form of guacamole—the list was endless.

With a vast world of choices now available to me, my postcollege busy life saw me eating every meal out and often on the go. I began to change my eating habits based on trends, not on food education. My day would start with Diet Coke and a whole-wheat egg wrap; twice a week, I'd skip the soda and treat myself to a Starbuck's white chocolate soy mocha and a buttered bagel or muffin. Always a salad for lunch, picked up near the office, and takeout on my way home for dinner, which would round out my day of eating. Once, when my parents were visiting, they opened my refrigerator and stared slack-jawed at the contents: a bottle of water and nail polish.

During these years, my Sunday night food ritual was my favorite. I'd head over to hang with a group of friends, order Chinese takeout, and each of us would grab a pint of our favorite ice cream. Together we'd eat in front of the TV while watching *Sex and the City*. This was as close to a family dinner as it got.

My relationship with food and what I was putting into my body was far from healthy.

I made my food choices based on what my friends were eating, what was inexpensive, what was readily available, and what I saw advertised on TV. Turns out, I was not alone. All around us we are being inundated with advertisements for food (mostly unhealthy choices), poor nutritional messages, and news that reports conflicting accounts of what proper nutrition actually is.[1] Not once did I ever associate how my body felt with what fueled it until I started to have stomach problems.

After lunch every day in the early 2000s, I'd end up hunched over my desk in pain. I went to a few different doctors, who suggested it might be stress. I even found an allergist thinking that maybe food allergies were to blame. Yet none of the tests yielded answers. After one particular appointment, the doctor asked about the kinds of food I was consuming before I started to feel the pain. Her response: "There are hundreds of preservatives out there. We can't test for all of them." With absolutely no advice other than "try eating something else," I left her office feeling more helpless than when I went in.

Those nights of packaged noodles from the corner store, a roasted chicken from the grocery, or sushi delivered from my favorite place down the street were full of who-knows-what ingredients. I never really stopped to think about it. According to the Dietary Guidelines Advisory Committee (DGAC), established jointly by the Secretaries of the U.S. Department of Health and Human Services (HHS) and the U.S. Department of Agriculture (USDA), "No matter where food is obtained, the diet quality of the U.S. population does not meet recommendations for vegetables, fruit, dairy, or whole grains, and exceeds recommendations for the nutrients sodium and saturated fat, refined grains, solid fats and added sugars leading to overconsumption."[2] So I started to keep a food journal to see whether I could figure out the issue myself. While the exercise didn't lead to any proof-positive answers, it did get me on the path to thinking about what I put in my body and how my body reacted to what I ate.

The scientific study of food and the effects it has on our bodies began quietly during the French Revolution in the late 1700s.[3] Prior to this, people experimented with foods and plants found in nature and through process of elimination determined which species were helpful or harmful. Today, as the field of nutrition continues to advance and new scientific understanding of our cellular composition is discovered, fresh information along with contradictory material arises, making it a vast, confusing field for the average person to understand. Our population relies on companies and health experts to tell us what foods will keep us healthy and which ones will make us ill. In this chapter, we'll explore the latest information available today, as well as gain an understanding of how eating plays a role in how you feel.

FOOD AS MEDICINE

The Food Pyramid, guaranteed to produce obesity in many people.[4]

—Dr. Andrew Weil, director, Arizona Center
for Integrative Medicine

A few years ago, a friend of mine went to an Ayurvedic doctor to get a third opinion on his health. He was young, always training for a new Iron Man competition, and had no apparent health issues. He was a strict vegetarian, bordering on vegan, yet he was always exhausted and felt like he had no energy. The doctor spoke to him at length about his work, relationships, and overall lifestyle, concluding that he needed to start eating meat. That night he went out for dinner, ordered chicken, and felt better than he had in years.

For me, giving up red meat lasted 10 years. One morning I woke up and my first thought was: today I will eat a steak. Much to the delight of my Argentine mother-in-law, she proudly cooked me a nice piece of meat that evening, and I ate it without any moral or physical issues. This feeling was much more than a craving and was probably the first time I had truly listened to my body when it came to food. Yet it wasn't until a few years later when I launched Pravassa and really started to pay attention to my wellness that I began to make significant changes to my eating habits.

Integrative medicine proponent Dr. Andrew Weil, author Michael Pollan, and chef Alice Waters (all champions of clean eating: eating whole minimally processed foods as close to their natural form as possible) have been spreading the message that what you put into your body plays an even bigger role in your overall wellness than you realize. Yet it is important to point out: **there is no one right way to eat.** Like sleep and exercise, how to get the most out of your diet will change as you age and as your lifestyle shifts. Yet the more you know about the food you are eating, the better equipped you are at determining which foods will fuel you and which will leave you regretting your choices.

There have been significant changes in the way we eat as a country in the last forty years. Everything from shifts within our nations work patterns to the food supply chain, how we study food in the field of nutrition to how we shop, has had influence over the ways in which we now eat. In 1990, the Nutrition Labeling and Education Act (NLEA) was passed, requiring all packaged foods to have a nutrition label and turning the consumer food education model on its head, and mandatory food education changes are still in full swing today. At the end of 2016, the FDA's calorie labeling, where calorie information will be clearly printed on the menus of all U.S. chain restaurants with 20 or more locations, will be a requirement. And by summer 2018, a new nutrition label, one that shows the amount of added sugar and vitamin D, will be on packaged food in grocery stores. With an abundance of nutritional information out there, why are chronic food-related diseases such as obesity and diabetes still on the rise?

Type 2 diabetes occurs when the body's blood sugar levels are elevated either due to lack of insulin or the body's inability to efficiently use that insulin. It used to be very rare. Since 1975, the percentage of Americans living with this disease has grown from 2.3% up to 7.2%.[5] This is a 313% increase in 40 years! This increase has resulted in 2.3 times higher medical expenditures, $176 billion in total that would be wiped out of our medical system in the United States if our population did not develop diabetes.[6] In late 2015, Temple University's Schools of Pharmacy and Medicine published a study in the journal of *Science Translational Medicine*, which found that after only a few days of overeating, early warning signs of type 2 diabetes can develop.[7]

As time passes between meals, our glucose levels drop, leaving us feeling weak, tired, and even fuzzy. The neuropeptide receptors in our brain act as a control for our hunger and regulate our survival mechanisms; these things signal the body that it's time to eat.[8] When we get hangry (hungry and angry), our body is signaling to us that our blood glucose levels are alarmingly low.

CHAPTER 6

Carbs, Protein, and Fat—What You Need to Know

Our bodies need a combination of carbohydrates, protein, and fat to thrive and keep our system healthy. There is no magical across-the-board combination for every person, so it's important to understand the basics of these nutrients in order to choose what's right for you.

> **Carbohydrates** fuel our muscles, provide energy for our brain, and help to manage stress. You'll get the most value out of eating complex carbohydrates such as vegetables and whole grains.
> **Protein** repairs the cells in our body and helps to generate new ones, controls inflammation, and carries vitamins through our digestive system. Beans, eggs, seafood, and lean meat such as a skinless chicken breast are the healthiest ways to get your protein.
> **Fats** get a bad rap, but if you're eating the right fats—healthy fats—it aids brain development, stabilizes insulin, and helps the body absorb vitamins. Look to consume avocados, coconut oil, olive oil, salmon, and nut butters (almond, cashew) for their healthy fats.

We can control this by consuming high-quality nutrients before we reach this state in ways such as healthy snacking—think nuts and vegetables. Instead, what we tend to do is reach for sugary snacks as a quick fix to up our glucose levels. This pattern wreaks havoc on our glycemic index and causes a chain reaction of inflammation, which leads to the crash-and-burn feeling associated with coming down from a sugar high.

Instead, if we eat to control our glycemic load by paying attention to a food's glycemic index (GI), a system of measurement that ranks how quickly food raises our blood glucose levels, we can create a balanced healthy diet. The goal of a low GI diet allows for fewer spikes to your internal system, enables the body to digest food at a slower rate, and helps to cut out cravings. You don't have to go crazy figuring out each food's GI, adding yet another item to your to-do list; instead use common sense and eat healthy. Items like white bread, ice cream, mangoes, and crackers have a high GI, while food such as sweet potatoes, brown rice, and carrots have a low GI.

If you suffer from chronic heartburn, chronic fatigue, high cholesterol, joint pain, and even Alzheimer's, your body may be suffering from internal inflammation (sort of like when you get a cut or injure a muscle). When we eat foods that cause internal stress, our systems respond with inflammation.[9] Our organs swell and sometimes develop a loss of function, which can inhibit tissue repair and the natural healing process. Do it often enough and our system starts to suffer chronic inflammation, leading to the above-mentioned aliments.

This inflammation has been shown to affect our physical health,[10] but it may also be associated with psychiatric disorders. According to Dr. Michael Berk, chair of psychiatry at Deakin University in Melbourne, Australia, "Unhealthy ('Western') patterns, high in red and processed meats, refined carbohydrate and other processed foods, [are] associated with increased inflammatory markers" and may play a role in bipolar disorder, schizophrenia, autism, and posttraumatic stress disorder.[11]

While starting on a diet of anti-inflammatory foods isn't a cure-all for our health problems, it has been shown to reduce organ stress and is often touted as a preventative measure when it comes to our physical health. Whole grains[12] and fermented foods[13] such as miso, kefir, kombucha, and sauerkraut have been the subjects of studies that have shown inflammation reduction. A 2001 study conducted by the Salk Institute for Biological Studies, a nonprofit research institute, found that flavonoids—red, blue, and purple naturally occurring pigments in fruits such as strawberries, blueberries, and plums—have shown to protect against Alzheimer's, dementia, and age-related memory loss.[14] And while more research needs to be conducted, other anti-inflammatory benefits from flavonoids include reduction in blood pressure, improvements in eyesight, and suppression in the spread of human cancer cells.[15]

The Mediterranean diet, high in plant-based foods and omega-3, consisting of some fish as well as healthy fats, is continuously cited as one of the healthiest lifestyle diets around. Not only has this way of eating been shown to reduce inflammation[16] and prostate cancer in men,[17] but the omega-3 fatty

Foods Play a Role in Inflammation

If we start to think about how food helps or hurts our internal system, it may be the catalyst for change that we need to improve the way we eat. Take note of how you feel the next time you eat these foods:

Foods that contribute to inflammation: alcohol, aspartame, dairy, fried foods, peanuts, refined sugar, and white bread.

Foods that are anti-inflammatory: almonds, beets, blueberries, broccoli, garlic, kale, kimchee, salmon, spinach, turmeric, and whole grains.

acids contribute to good heart health and can provide protection against reduced plasticity and impaired learning after a traumatic brain injury.[18] Sounds like it's time to up your intake of extra virgin olive oil and wild-caught salmon!

Fasting and detoxing are internal cleansing techniques that have been used for centuries, going back to primitive cultures for religious reasons, and are still prevalent today: Jews fast for Yom Kippur, Muslims for Ramadan, and Catholics for Lent. These forms of food restriction have also been used to treat illness, lose weight, and restore balance to the body. Our digestive system, made up of large, bulky organs, is always working. Overnight we give the system respite, allowing it to use energy for digestion and healing purposes, before we break that fast again in the morning.

Short-term fasting, 1 to 3 days, is often prescribed as a home remedy to battle colds and flus, to reduce internal inflammation, and to help break food addictions. Clinical psychologist Douglas Lisle says his "patients have had the most success in breaking food addictions with therapeutic, water-only fasting in medically supervised settings."[19] I myself use fasting as a "reset" technique whenever I travel. An airplane is the perfect place to rest your digestive system instead of asking it to work overtime by feeding it unhealthy plane food. Not only have the effects helped me significantly reduce my jet lag symptoms, but it also reduces insulin spikes and rebalances blood sugar levels,[20]

Eliminate These Food Triggers

Want to know how food affects your body? Many integrative healthcare professionals advocate for the elimination diet, a way of eating first proposed by Dr. Albert Rowe in 1941.[1] Rowe presented guidelines on how to eliminate foods from your diet if you had allergies in order to cure yourself. Today's common food intolerances and the subject of many modern-day elimination diets are:

- Cow's milk
- Eggs
- Corn
- MSG (Monosodium Glutamate)

- Peanuts
- Shellfish
- Soy
- Wheat

NOTE

1. Rowe, Albert H., *Elimination Diets and the Patient's Allergies: A Handbook of Allergy* (Philadelphia: Lea & Febiger, 1941).

meaning that I start to crave healthier nutrient-dense food when it's time to eat again.

If fasting to eliminate toxins in the body is not something that interests you, sweating is another perfectly natural way to achieve similar results. Aside from exercise, spending time in a sauna or steam room is highly recommended to eliminate uric acid.[21] When you use heat to dilate blood vessels, circulation is sped up and the pores in the skin open allowing the body to sweat. Sweating is a detoxification method that reduces the workload of both the kidneys and liver, whose main job is to filter toxins out of the blood stream. Heading to the sauna is my other go-to method of reset when I check into a new hotel. Just remember, both time in an airplane and a sauna are dehydrating. In order to stay healthy, you need to replenish your system with lots and lots of water.

When it comes to looking at food as medicine, the hard-charging high-stress lives we lead also deplete our bodies of important vitamins and minerals that we need to optimally function. For example, vitamin A is good for the healthy development of teeth and skin, vitamin C for strengthening blood vessels, and folic acid for cell renewal. Yet when we reach for nutrient-poor food, we are depriving our bodies of the exact things they need to stay healthy.

Low levels of vitamin D, which are widespread among Western populations, have been linked to osteoporosis and cancer[22] as well as anxiety and depression.[23] Having a magnesium deficiency due to stress or the foods we eat not only impairs the body by presenting with physical symptoms such as leg cramps and tension headaches,[24] but also causes a chain reaction and can lead to a loss of vitamins B2 and B6.[25] This list goes on.

Many doctors recommend taking supplements to counteract vitamin and mineral deficiencies, yet many do not. This big divide in treatment approaches is due to the fact that dietary supplement manufacturers and distributors are not required to obtain regulatory approval or perform clinical tests before marketing their products. With debates to be had on both sides of this argument, Dr. Weil has said it best: "Vitamins, minerals and other supplements won't compensate for a poor diet, but they can help fill nutritional gaps in a good one."[26] So to make sure you're giving your body a great base to start from, it's important to have a diet that varies in foods (fish, nuts, seeds, fruits, vegetables, protein, whole grains), textures (crunchy, soft, smooth) and colors (eat the rainbow). If diet and exercise still leave you feeling like something is off, consult a medical professional to see whether a vitamin or mineral deficiency might be to blame.

DO YOU KNOW THE MUFFIN MAN?

> *Make your calories count, but don't count your calories.*[27]
>
> —Jared Koch, Clean Plates founder

TV's *Biggest Loser*, Internet pop-ups ads, spam emails touting weight loss supplements—big business is sending us a message: it's time to lose weight. A total of 2.1 billion people, nearly 30%

of the world's population, are overweight,[28] with 155 million living in the United States.[29] If lumped together, this number would visually represent everyone living west of the eastern United States. A recent study published in *Obesity Research & Clinical Practice* found that it's harder for adults today to maintain the same weight as 30 years ago, even when eating the same levels of food and exercising.[30]

Well that sucks. Ask anyone, even yourself, and I'm betting most people would be more than happy to shed a few pounds from their current frame.

How did we get here? Jennifer Kuk, professor of kinesiology and health science at Toronto's York University who worked on the *Obesity* study, thinks that exposure to chemicals, use of prescription selective serotonin reuptake inhibitors (SSRIs), changes in our gut bacteria, and artificial sweeteners might all be to blame.[31] The food we eat is a collection of molecules that we digest and our bodies break down to use as fuel. And while a calorie is a calorie, we gain weight whether we eat healthy or not.

But not all calories carry equal nutrients, which is a huge factor when looking at overall body health and the health of our organs. Consuming too many nutrient-deficient calories through poor food decisions not only leads to weight gain, but also alters our body's ability over time to regulate weight and metabolism.[32] In 2008, medical costs associated with obesity carried a hefty cost in the United States: $147 billion.[33] Obesity contributes to everything from heart disease to diabetes to high blood pressure to liver disease, chronic conditions that often need to be managed with medication and frequent doctor visits. Obesity has been studied in its relationship to the brain and the long-term effects it presents. A study in Australia linked obesity to an increase in depression later in life,[34] and scientists at Kent State in Ohio have shown that obesity in midlife is associated with an increased risk of dementia down the road.[35]

Doctors at Weill Cornell Medical Center in the United States have shown how overeating on the typical American diet actually changes the brain and the way it regulates metabolism.[36] Hence, the constant reminders to lose weight via advertisements touting a new fad diet, supplement, or fitness regime, all of which promise to be the magic weight loss cure. And as a nation, we're buying! Nearly, two-thirds of Americans[37] are currently trying to lose weight by cutting calories, fats, and sugar from their diet. And cutting calories works—at first. It's a simple math problem: when you decrease the amount of calories you intake, your weight drops in relationship. Yet if this is the only change you make, it is not sustainable—New Year's Resolutions, anyone?

In 2009, the National Weight Control Registry conducted an experiment on calorie restriction. The results: 97 women lost an average of 27 pounds per person.[38] Yet, each and every person returned to their old eating habits after the experiment, regaining some if not all of the weight they had shed. However, if you approach calorie restriction as a lifestyle change, looking at all parts of your life that contribute to the way you consume food, then a long-term change may in fact succeed. Turning toward a more conscious eating plan, one that looks at the kind of calories you consume and when and how you consume them, will help disrupt old eating habits and is a path that nutritionists and dieticians alike are turning toward, hoping that their message resonates.

A common myth you can set aside today is that skipping breakfast will help you to kick-start a weight loss cycle. People who typically skip breakfast are more likely to be overweight, as skipping this first meal of the day impairs fasting lipids and creates insulin sensitivity, which can lead to weight gain.[39] Instead, by starting your day with a meal that is high in protein, you set the tone for your food intake, stemming cravings and keeping yourself full. By eating your dinner in front of the TV, you're setting yourself up for weight gain too, as your mind is focused on the program, not on your food. In fact, "the more distracting the (TV) program is the more you will eat," says Dr. Aner Tal of the Cornell Food and Brain Lab.[40]

Obesity, which affects so many people, is a long-term imbalance between energy intake and expenditure. A lot of knowledge in this area comes from a 2006 NASA study on bedrest. After a couple of days of nonactivity, the body's metabolism becomes inflexible.[41] Once you start moving again, the metabolism responds. By choosing sedentary behaviors over exercise and eating junk food sitting in front of the TV over and over again, you are reinforcing poor habits around food, which leads to packing on the pounds.

FEED YOUR SOUL

> *One cannot think well, love well, sleep well, if one has not dined well.*[42]

—Virginia Woolf

10 years old. Feeling sad = have chocolate to cheer up.
13 years old. It's your birthday = start the special day with cake for breakfast.
16 years old. Just won a huge volleyball match – eat frozen yogurt to celebrate.
23 years old. Stressed out = grab a pint of ice cream as dinner.

These are plot points on my emotional food timeline. Many of us have learned to manage our emotions this way, creating deep-seated issues which tie food to self-worth and happiness and act as roadblocks when we try to lose weight or change our eating habits.

We need to eat to live; therefore, any eating behaviors we've developed—feeding our happy, sad, accomplished, failed selves—are much more difficult to change than any other addiction. Why? According to clinical psychologist Tian Dayton, "Using food to deaden stressed out or uncomfortable emotions, in much the same way as an alcoholic might use liquor, is still gaining acceptance as a coping mechanism."[43] Currently, there is a lack of a cohesive definition for food addiction within the medical community. Yet when Dr. Ashley Gearhardt studied eating disorders in her work for Yale University, she found that 57% of the patients she examined fell within the Yale Food Addiction Scale, exhibiting higher levels of depression, emotion dysregulation, and lower self-esteem,[44] all of which can happen with long-term exposure to an unhealthy diet.

Binge eating disorder (BED) is one area of food addiction that has been extensively studied and is something many people exhibit signs of but don't realize. BED is characterized as consuming large amounts of food at various times and reveals itself as eating when depressed or bored or eating until you are physically uncomfortable and then feeling disgusted or guilty after eating so much.[45] When food is consumed in this way, it leads the body to develop unhealthy associations, and many people return to food to cope with the negative feelings, creating a cycle that is hard to break.

Both food and drug cravings exhibit similar patterns of addiction in the neural mechanism of the brain. Rats that are fed diets based on sugar, fat, and processed foods exhibit the behavioral trademarks of addiction such as tolerance, withdrawal, and continued use despite the negative consequences.[46] A food addiction, such as overeating, can make you feel lethargic and physically too full, can lead to harsh personal judgments, and can even trigger painful emotions.[47] Yet even if we feel this way, we often continue the cycle of self-medication with food.

When the body has low blood sugar, it can cause mood swings and depression. Yet stuffing yourself with refined carbs and sugar (so good while eating them) spikes the body's glucose levels, which can leave you feeling tired and cranky once you crash. Changing what you put in your body to be more healthful not only reduces our emotional reactivity, but also puts us in a better state of emotional health to begin with.[48]

If food can be used to self-regulate our negative emotions, it stands to reason it can be used to produce positive emotions too. Eating dark chocolate has long been a go-to to help reduce negative feelings, and while studies have shown that the oligomeric PC compound in dark chocolate does have a positive effect, when you factor in the sugar and milk that make up the rest of the chocolate bar, the effects are short-lived, often disappearing after 3 minutes.[49] While not as sexy as chocolate, omega-3 fatty acids, long touted for their positive effects on cardiovascular health, may be the better choice as they may play a role in the treatment of mood disorders such as depression.[50]

Studies have suggested that long-term exposure to unhealthy dietary habits independently predisposes one to depression over the course of a lifetime.[51] Currently, a study is underway in Australia which looks at the relationship between diet and mental health. Researchers are delving into the field to find out if nutritional deficiencies associated with depression can be remedied by overhauling one's diet or by taking nutritional supplements.[52]

In chapter 2, we looked at how food and sleep are intertwined and how eating a diet high in inflammatory foods can lead to

Healthy Behaviors to Refocus Your Emotions

We turn to food to manage all sorts of emotions. What if we were able to learn to replace those habits with healthier alternatives? Next time you feel yourself reaching for food to lift your mood, try one of these options instead and note the difference.

Refocus your attention—Breathe, meditate, or think about an upcoming vacation or a vacation you just returned from to focus on a happier place.

Get into downward dog—Yoga, running, or any other physical activity gets you out of your head and into your body.

Drink tea—If you feel compelled to put something in your mouth, try this hot, soothing, low-calorie ritual.

Phone a friend—Having someone listen to you will rid your body of overwhelming emotions and will provide a support system that isn't linked to food.

more vivid dreams and disrupt sleep patterns. When the sleep cycle is disrupted, there is a greater tendency to snack. Often snack food increases our intake of fat and sweets in order to give us the rush of energy we need to stay awake.[53] If we look at our digestive system as a mirror to our state of mind, when we skip meals due to stress, eat late at night to help get over a hard day, or dine on food with poor nutritional quality, we are setting ourselves up for emotional eating. Instead, understanding your emotional reactivity to food is one of the things that will contribute toward a positive change in your eating habits.

YOU'RE ALREADY SWEET ENOUGH

Sugar. Give me sugar. And water. More. More.[54]

—Vincent D'Onofrio's character,
Edgar, in *Men in Black*

I love sugar. I like how it tastes. I like how it feels in my mouth. I like the boost of energy it gives me immediately after I consume it. I am addicted to sugar. So, it should come as no surprise that once I started paying attention to the labels on my food, I saw that sugar appeared as an additive in almost everything I was eating. The whole grain bread I had for breakfast—added sugar. The fat-free dressing on my salad at lunch—added sugar. The protein smoothie for my afternoon snack—added sugar. The dried banana chips I ate after dinner—added sugar. According to award-winning journalist and professor of journalism at UC Berkeley, Michael Pollan, "We are biologically designed to like food high in sugar, fat, and salt because of when food was scarce. Now [these additives] are abundant and our biology is mismatched with what is occurring in the food environment."[55]

David Ludwig, a professor of pediatrics and nutrition at Harvard University and a researcher at Boston Children's Hospital, notes that our bodies seek out sugar when we are stressed because it comforts us immediately.[56] When we eat sugar it affects the same neurological pathways as narcotics, repeatedly elevating our dopamine levels, which control our brain's reward center.[57] Yet the more sugar we consume over time, the greater tolerance we build up to its effects, meaning eventually that we need more and more sugar to receive the same "high."

You may be aware of the famous French study that was published in 2007, whose research showed that sweeteners are more addictive than cocaine when tested on rats. In the study, rats were allowed to choose between water sweetened with saccharin and intravenous cocaine. Ninety-four percent of the rats preferred the sweetener.[58] Since this research was released, the studies on sugar and its addictive nature have intensified leading some in the medical community to believe that sugar damages the body in the same manner as drug abuse. In 2016, researchers have suggested that treating sugar addiction with varenicline, commonly known as Chantix and marketed as a smoking cessation aid, may help reduce the body's need for sugar consumption.[59]

Aside from possible addiction, we reach for sugar because it's the path of least resistance. Remember reading about decision fatigue in chapter 2? This is something that the body and brain experience throughout the day as we grow tired. At the end of the day, we look for shortcuts in all areas, including nourishment, which has us reaching for sugar to quickly restore energy. We end up playing out a cycle, which becomes a Catch-22; we turn toward sugar to boost glucose and restore willpower and self-control, which is supposed to help us resist the sugar we just reached for. Each time we do this, we're reinforcing a bad habit and spiking/crashing our blood sugar. Instead we should be eating healthier foods that provide a steady, even supply of glucose so we don't find ourselves reaching for the easiest option.

The American Heart Association recommends no more than 6 teaspoons of sugar a day for the average woman and no more than 9 teaspoons for the average man.[60] Yet, the average American is consuming 22 teaspoons per day[61]—almost 3 times the recommended amount. So where is our sugar intake coming from, and why is it so out of whack with the recommended daily guidelines? "There is a lot of hidden sugar in our food supply,"[62] Dr. Frank Hu, a member of the Dietary Guidelines Advisory Committee, told the New York Times in an article about limited sugar consumption.

A lot of the foods we eat have naturally occurring sugar. Fruits, vegetables, and even milk are examples, whose makeup is accompanied by other nutrients such as fiber, vitamins, minerals, and water. The body needs these other nutrients to function optimally and to help the body to processes the sugar we are consuming. But the excess sugar we eat is not typically naturally occurring. Instead, it is estimated that 74% of the packaged foods sold in the United States contain added sugar.[63] Currently our nutrition labels show sugar as one line item of ingredients; it does not differentiate between natural and added sugar. This will change in 2018 when the updated nutrition label breaks out added sugar as a separate line item. In the meantime, it's up to each of us to decipher the "good" from the "bad" sugars. Added sugar can be labeled as agave, brown sugar, cane sugar, corn syrup, fructose, dextrose, fruit juice concentrate, glucose, honey, maltose, and molasses, among others.

Sugar causes inflammation, weight gain, tooth decay, and type 2 diabetes. Most U.S. adults know this, but are still consuming way too much of it. Adults who consume 25% or more of their

Why You Need to Stop Drinking Soda Now

Research suggests that our bodies are less aware of excessive intake of calories and sugar when they are delivered in liquid form.[1] In 2012, New York City mayor Michael Bloomberg made national headlines when he called for a ban on soda and other sugary drinks larger than 16 ounces. While public health advocates praised his proposal, the courts struck down the ban, so it never went into effect. Regardless of your political stance on this proposed ban, here's what you need to know about soda:

- A single 12-ounce can of sugar-sweetened soda contains up to 40 grams (around 10 teaspoons) of free sugars (sugars added during the production process).[2]
- A 64-ounce Double Gulp from 7-Eleven comes with a whopping 44 teaspoons of sugar.[3]
- 92% of U.S. adults experience tooth decay; a major source of this problem is sugar found in soda.[4]
- People who drink more than 4 cups of soda per day are 30% more likely to develop depression than those who don't drink soda.[5]
- Worldwide, 184,000 deaths a year are attributable to sugar-sweetened beverages.[6]
- Women who drink more than two servings of sugary beverages every day have a 40% higher risk of heart attacks or death from heart disease than women who rarely drink sugary beverages.[7]

NOTES

1. Moss, Michael, *Salt Sugar Fat: How the Food Giants Hooked Us* (New York: Random House, 2013).

2. World Health Organization, "WHO Calls on Countries to Reduce Sugars Intake among Adults and Children," March 4, 2015. www.who.int /mediacentre/news/releases/2015/sugar-guideline/en/

3. Moss, Michael, *Salt Sugar Fat: How the Food Giants Hooked Us* (New York: Random House, 2013).

4. Sheiham, Aubrey, W. Philip, and T. James, "A Reappraisal of the Quantitative Relationship Between Sugar Intake and Dental Caries: The Need for New Criteria for Developing Goals for Sugar Intake," *BMC Public Health*. DOI: 10.1186/1471-2458-14-863

5. American Academy of Neurology, "Hold the Diet Soda? Sweetened Drinks Linked to Depression, Coffee Tied to Lower Risk," January 8, 2013.

6. Singh, Gitanjali M., et al., "Estimated Global, Regional, and National Disease Burdens Related to Sugar-Sweetened Beverage Consumption in 2010," American Heart Association, 2015. DOI: 10.1161/CIRCULATIONAHA.114.010636

7. Fung, T. T., V. Malik, K. M. Rexrode, J. E. Manson, W. C. Willett, and F. B. Hu, "Sweetened Beverage Consumption and Risk of Coronary Heart Disease in Women," *Am J Clin Nutr* 89 (2009): 1037–42.

daily calories in sugar (over 500 calories based on a 2,000/day calorie diet) are nearly three times more likely to die of heart disease than those who only ingest 10% of their daily calories from sugar.[64] "Many problems get solved when you get off the sugar train,"[65] writes Amy Shah, and she's not the only medical professional who thinks this way. "We have solid evidence that keeping intake of free sugars to less than 10% of total energy intake reduces the risk of obesity, tooth decay, and being overweight," says Francesco Branca, director of WHO's Department of Nutrition for Health and Development.[66]

The year 2015 was a big one for sugar, as guidelines for use and government policy changes around the world put these crystals on notice. In March, the World Health Organization released new daily recommendations, which said people should reduce their sugar intake to less than 10% of their overall diet in order to halt the rise in diabetes and obesity.[67] Ten months later the U.S. Food and Drug Administration followed suit and placed the same recommended cap, 12.5 teaspoons per day,[68] or a can of Coke, on our diet for the first time ever. Not even six months after that, the U.S. Department of Agriculture and Department of Health and Human Services joined the movement and recommended the same sugar limit, which is a huge step as the guides created by this department impact what goes into school lunches and lays out the way government programs promote healthy diets.[69]

> **Best Ways to Kick Your Sugar Habit Now**
>
> - Eat nutrient-dense filling food: whole grains, lean protein, and vegetables.
> - Be mindful of the foods you eat and how your body reacts to them. Cut out or cut down on items that make you feel bloated or stuffed-up or give you a headache.
> - Stop eating foods with high sugar content: barbecue sauce, ketchup, cereal, and muffins.
> - Manage stress by blowing off steam in a healthy way.
> - Work out regularly by getting your heart pumping for at least 20 minutes every day.
> - Get quality, uninterrupted sleep every night to help kick any cravings.

Like any addiction, it's hard to break free of sugar cold-turkey. Instead, it's much easier—and healthier—to feed that fix by turning toward naturally occurring sugars. Ditch the soda, cereal, and ice cream from your routine and instead reach for fruit or put a little honey in your tea. After a few weeks you'll not only notice the difference, but if you return to your old eating habits, you'll be surprised to find that the foods you used to like so much don't taste like anything but heaps and heaps of sugar. Trust me, I've tried it!

EAT REAL FOOD

> *Cheap food is an illusion. The real cost of the food is paid somewhere. And if it isn't paid at the cash register, it's charged to your health.*[70]
>
> —Michael Pollan

In 2001, Americans were given a glimpse into the U.S. fast-food industry when a book, and later a movie, called *Fast Food Nation* was published by investigative journalist Eric Schlosser.

The book became a catalyst and opened the door for national conversations surrounding food safety, animal welfare, and obesity, paving the way for other influential authors and chefs such as Michael Pollan and Jamie Oliver as well as filmmakers like Morgan Spurlock and his *Super Size Me* documentary to continue the dialog. Today, you can't get online without seeing a headline relating to food, whether it's about GMOs, organic food, sustainability, outbreaks of food-borne illnesses, or the cost of all of this to our wallets.

While there is no legal definition for processed food, items produced in a laboratory with input and tinkering from scientists clearly fall under this label. For years, the U.S. government has subsidized crops such as corn, soy, wheat, and rice, which help to keep prices low and production high, supplying food giants with these ingredients. Pulitzer Prize-winning author Michael Moss sat down with U.S. scientists and food executives for his 2013 book *Salt Sugar Fat: How the Food Giants Hooked Us* to learn more. During the course of his research, Moss interviewed an experimental psychologist from Harvard, Howard Moskowitz, who coined the term "bliss point," a subtle tweaking in food formulas to a point that perfects the greatest amount of crave and helps products sell.[71] By purchasing government subsidized ingredients and altering the food's bliss point to sell more products, food industries began to see their biggest profits on the items they processed.[72]

Interestingly enough, Moss learned that both the scientists and food executives employed by these food giants "don't eat their own products, because they know better. They know about the addictive properties of sugar, salt and fat."[73] The way that we've been eating for the last 40 years has created a long-term imbalance between our energy intake and expenditure, increasing consumption of more energy-dense, nutrient-poor foods containing high levels of sugar and saturated fats,[74] all of which contribute to our health problems. It has caused a backlash, and today, the movement toward eating healthier is gaining ground. Consumers have access to more and more information about the ways in which food is grown, harvested, and shipped, and they are making choices with their wallet.

About Those Food Labels

Prior to 1990, packaged food in the United States was not required to bear a nutrition label. Yet during the passing of the Nutrition Labeling and Education Act (NLEA), the government agreed that if the food contained an insignificant amount of ingredients with respect to the overall nutritional value, then those things did not need to be labeled.[1] Additionally, in a move to appease food lobbyists, the NLEA allowed health claims such as "high fiber," "low fat," and "light" to be used on packaged food as long as these claims were consistent with agency regulations.[2] So, are we getting real nutritional information or marketing spin? Again, it's up to us to decide. Here are a few things to keep in mind the next time you read that nutrition label:

- Ingredients are listed in order of the highest percentage contained in the food.
- Foods that are "fortified" or "enriched" with vitamins and minerals have these nutrients added into the food product after it has lost these components during processing.[3]
- Milk and meats that are not labeled "no antibiotics" or "no hormones" can contain both, either from injections to the animal or via the food the animals are fed.[4]
- While still under review by the FDA, food dyes which are derived from petroleum, such as Red 40, Yellow 5, and Yellow 6, have been associated with behavioral problems in children.[5]

NOTES

1. 101st Congress (1989-1990), "H.R.3562—Nutrition Labeling and Education Act of 1990," House—Energy and Commerce. 11/8/1990 Became Public Law No: 101-535.
2. US Food and Drug Administration, "Nutritional Labeling and Education Act (NLEA) Requirements (8/94-2/95)." http://www.fda.gov/iceci/inspections/inspectionguides/ucm074948.htm

3. Medical Dictionary. S. v., "enriched food," Retrieved April 1, 2016 from http://medical-dictionary.thefreedictionary.com/enriched+food
4. United States Department of Agriculture, "Meat and Poultry Labeling Terms," August 2015, www.fsis.usda.gov/wps/portal/fsis/topics/food-safety-education/get-answers/food-safety-fact-sheets/food-labeling/meat-and-poultry-labeling-terms/meat-and-poultry-labeling-terms
5. Potera, Carol, "Diet and Nutrition: The Artificial Food Dye Blues," *Environmental Health Perspectives* 118, 10 (October 2010): A428. DOI: 10.1289/Ehp.118-A428

The changes in our dietary habits over the past decade have manifested in people eating higher-fiber, nutrient-dense foods, replacing saturated fats with omega-3s.[75] Consumers are reading more labels, asking more questions about additives, educating themselves about free-range and grass-fed animals, and looking into what it means to eat a sustainable diet. Consumers advocating for organic food are showing that they are very willing to pay a premium for it.[76] Even the Obama administration got into the act when it brought back the White House garden after a 60-year absence as a way to educate the public about the role food consumption plays in our health.

Food manufacturers are listening too. Companies are moving away from artificial ingredients, and food products are being reformulated to eliminate or reduce the sugar, cholesterol, trans fats, saturated fats, and sodium in favor of fiber and protein.[77] Packaged foods now feature healthy call-outs, and in the past few years, sales of "natural" and "organic" foods have grown almost 28%.[78] Yet Michael Pollan warns against these claims. He says the "healthiest food is real food—it doesn't make any health claims—it doesn't come in fancy packages."[79] And to his point he's right, but in this era of information overload, many of which is confusing, we often need someone to tell us which foods are "good" and which ones are "bad"—hence all the marketing.

"Everyone is convinced that the government subsidies that support processed food need to be shifted over to fresh fruits and vegetables or it's going to continue to be hard for people who want to eat better,"[80] Michael Moss told *Time Magazine*. Until this happens, it is going to be up to each individual to determine how to eat better for themselves.

IT LIVES IN YOUR BELLY, BABY

"Is your gut healthy?" Five years ago, I could not imagine anyone asking me this question, let alone it being the subject line for article after article that has suddenly started to appear in my Facebook feed. The increased interest and development in gut health, due to technological advances in DNA sequencing and the creation of the Human Microbiome Project (HMP), a research organization that began in 2008 with a $150 million budget to conduct a 5-year study,[81] seems to be an inescapable topic when it comes to one's overall well-being. "Ten years ago, microbiomes were hardly on the map. Last year, 25,000 papers contained the term."[82] This statement, which recently appeared in a Google Hangout session on understanding the microbiome, underscores that the topic of gut health has exploded to become the latest talked-about medical advance today.

The Center for Ecogenetics and Environmental Health tells us that the microbiome is genetic material (bacteria, fungi, protozoa, and viruses) that lives on and inside the human body.[83] This material helps to digest our food, regulate our immune system, protect against invading bacteria, and produce the vitamins that we need to stay healthy. The microbiome, not generally recognized until the late 1990s, shows that humans are made up of more than 100 trillion microbes, the majority of which live in our large intestine.[84] Since the gut microbiome has begun to be studied, talk of prebiotics and probiotics, as well as how they affect our diet, has entered the layman's lexicon in full force. Before I talk about the effects of these "biotics on our gut," let's understand what they are:

Prebiotics are nondigestible plant fibers that live in the large intestine and beneficially affect the body by selectively stimulating the growth and/or activity of the body's gut bacteria,[85] essentially providing food for the probiotics to thrive off. Some examples of food that carry prebiotics are bananas, honey, onions, and garlic.

Probiotics are live microorganisms that benefit the body by stimulating the growth of other microorganisms and improve the nutritional and microbial balance in the intestinal tract.[86] These live active cultures are what food companies call out in their marketing and they can be found in items such as yogurt, kefir, kimchi, miso, and tempeh.

"The majority of ingredients in the industrially produced foods consumed in the West are absorbed in the upper part of small intestine and thus of limited benefit to the microbiota. Lack of proper nutrition for microbiota is a major factor chronically elevating inflammation,"[87] writes Stig Bengmark, emeritus professor at University College in London. Therefore, as doctors and scientists begin to understand how our body's microbiota grows, so will the ways to treat and change it, starting with how we eat.

A 2009 study conducted at the University of Pennsylvania School of Medicine[88] found that when switching mice to a high-fat diet, they observed changes in the gut microbiome, which begs the question: if we change our diet, can we improve our overall health? If the answer is yes, then that means in the future we might be able to predict which foods will have good or bad impact on our bodies based on our individual microbiome. Currently, fermented foods, which carry the highest amounts of live active cultures found in our food supply today, have been shown to positively influence our gut bacteria.[89] While there is still confusion around the dosages and duration in which they need to be ingested to achieve desired results, it is clear that there is some positive value for our bodies here.

A growing number of studies[90] have shown links between our microbiomes and numerous autoimmune diseases such as diabetes, rheumatoid arthritis, muscular dystrophy, and multiple sclerosis, which excites researchers with the possibility of not only understanding these diseases better, but also that manipulating our microbiome could be used to treat the diseases themselves. Dr. Emeran Mayer, a professor of medicine and psychiatry at the University of California, Los Angeles, told NPR's *Morning Edition* that he believes "our gut microbes affect what goes on in our brains."[91] Researchers have been looking into this link as well and have discovered that by altering the microbiota in mice, they find changes happen in brain chemistry and behavior.[92]

While all of this is exciting stuff, scientists and doctor alike agree that the field of microbiomes is just beginning to be

How to Keep Your Belly Happy When Traveling

When I travel, the first thing that usually acts up is my stomach. Whether it's Bali belly, Delhi belly, or just bloating, changing diet, time zones, and water intake, any and all of it can leave the digestive system protesting. Try these tips to increase your chances of a happy belly:

- **Don't eat on the airplane**—Fasting on the plane rests your digestive system, giving it a clean slate upon arrival.
- **Pack a probiotic**—While a full understanding of the health benefits of probiotics is lacking at the moment, the ones that have been clinically studied thus far have shown positive effects on irritable bowel syndrome and diarrhea.[1] Talk to your health professional about which ones will improve your gut health.
- **Drink a lot of water**—Water stimulates every cell in our body, and generally we don't drink enough of it on a normal day. Traveling dehydrates your system, so in order to feed our cells and promote healing, we need more water.
- **Take activated charcoal**—Never travel without this all-around toxin absorber that helps prevent gas and bloating.
- **Start your day with gut-healthy food**—Miso soup in Japan, yogurt in Europe, or bananas in Central America will all boost inner ecology and help to digest the rest of your food throughout the day.

NOTE

1. Brown, Alan, "Microbial Manifesto: The Global Push to Understand the Microbiome," March 2, 2016, *Google Hangout* session, transcribed at http://www.livescience.com/53916-understanding-life-means-understanding-microbes.html

understood. Right now the surface is just being scratched as to how all of this contributes to the gut's long-term stability toward health and illness. Right now the tests and experiments being performed are at the forefront in the field of research, which means brand new discoveries could be just around the corner.

YOUR FOOD FUTURE

Diet has the distinction of being the only major determinant of health that is completely under your control.[93]

—Dr. Andrew Weil

Are you a vegetarian? Do you follow the Paleo diet? Are most of your calories ingested in liquid form? Do you eat most of your meals on the go or in front of the TV? The Advisory Committee for Dietary Guidelines believes that individual nutritional behaviors and other health-related lifestyle behaviors are strongly influenced by our personal, social, organizational, and environmental contexts,[94] meaning that everything around you, including the company you keep, influences the ways in which you eat.

If we've already established that healthy, nutrient-dense calories keep hunger at bay, help to maintain stable blood sugar levels, and keep us full, why do we keep reaching for high-calorie, nutrient-deficient foods? Aside from the fact that they've been engineered to taste great, a large portion of this answer can be attributed to food marketing. Temple Northup said, "Those who watch a lot of television tend to have a more unhealthy diet than those who watch less. Within advertising, most foods are nutritionally deficient while entertainment programming depicts characters frequently snacking on unhealthy foods and rarely eating a balanced meal. If these are the messages, those who watch a lot of them may become less able to determine what is healthy."[95]

How many times have you watched your favorite TV show at night and seen a commercial for a hot, sizzling new menu item at the nearest chain restaurant? While this commercial might not cause you to take immediate action, it may change your spending habits tomorrow to curb the craving. Or worse, it could have your kids begging you to take them to try this latest concoction.

Food You Need to Stop Eating Today

Want to make a difference in your mood, weight, or sugar cravings? Cut out these foods today:

Fruit juice cocktails—Fruit juice on its own may contain much-needed vitamins, but the versions sold in stores are often watered down with added sugar and contain a small amount of actual juice.[1] Plus you are not getting any of the fiber or phytonutrient benefits that come with eating an actual apple or orange.

Venti anything at Starbucks—Would you like some coffee with your sugar? A 2016 research study found that signature mixed coffee and chai drinks at Starbucks have between 10 and 25 teaspoons of sugar per serving, all of which exceed the daily recommended amounts of sugar.[2]

Donuts—These deep-fried balls of sugar are tasty, but they pack on weight, as each serving is full of empty calories and trans fat, which raises cholesterol and increases your risk of heart disease and stroke.[3]

Margarine—Full of trans fat, even if it claims not to be, butter is a better option, as the saturated fat is a natural alternative.

Processed meat—These goodies can be purchased from your deli counter and include things like sausage, smoked meats, or bacon. A 2013 study found that these preservative and sodium laden foods have been linked to heart disease and stomach cancer.[4]

Soda—Sugar, tooth decay, death, plus plenty of reasons above to say goodbye to soda for good.

NOTES

1. Jacobsen, Maryann Tomovich, "Juices: The Best and Worst for Your Health," *WebMD*, May 2014. http://www.webmd.com/diet/ss/slideshow -juice-wars

2. Action on Sugar, "Shocking Amount of Sugar Found in Many Hot Fla-voured Drinks," February 17, 2016. www.actiononsugar.org/news%20centre/surveys%20/2016/170865.html#sthash.5fr3he4u.dpuf

3. American Heart Association, "Trans Fats," October 2015. www.heart.org/heartorg/healthyliving/fatsandoils/fats101/trans-fats_ucm_301120_article.jsp#.vyy_saodfbc

4. Rohrmann, Sabine, et al., "Meat Consumption and Mortality—Results from the European Prospective Investigation into Cancer and Nutrition," *BMC Medicine* 11, 63 (2013). DOI: 10.1186/1741-7015-11-63

Seventeen percent of U.S. kids between the ages of 6 and 11 are obese; these overweight children are more likely to develop high blood pressure, high cholesterol, and type 2 diabetes.[96] This is why it is important to start teaching our children healthy food habits from an early age. With food education on the rise, younger generations are looking to be more involved in their food choices, although they shy away from the complexity of understanding the entire system. They instead gravitate toward a simple and easy-to-appreciate supply chain: farm-to-table.

And it seems the groundwork we've begun to lay is work-ing. The upcoming Generation Z, newborns to 23 year olds, is the healthiest generation yet, taking the wellness lifestyle cultivated by millennials to the next level. The 2015 Nielsen's *Global Health and Wellness Survey* showed that of the youngest consumers with buying power, 41% would be willing to pay a premium for healthier foods.[97] People of every generation are now seeking out food that tastes good, doesn't cost a fortune, and has ingredients that have been shown to keep us healthy. This movement toward coveting more healthy, affordable options has caused the fast food chains to take notice and adapt to hold onto market share. Chick-fil-A has introduced a kale-based salad to their menu, McDonald's now offers oatmeal for breakfast, and Subway introduced a rotisserie-style chicken, the chain's first protein choice raised without antibiotics. And while I don't advocate getting your healthy food from these establishments, it's definitely a step in the right direction.

I truly believe that good health begins with what you feed your body. This was the hardest chapter for me to write because I am still practicing, tweaking, and coming to terms with my own food habits. I used writing this chapter as a catalyst to make some significant changes, which I have known for a year that I needed to make, but trotted out every excuse not to make them. Now with something to hold me accountable, you as the reader, I made a decision. It was time to take that final push and change my relationship to food by cutting out added sugar. The goal was to sit and eat each meal mindfully at my kitchen table, significantly reduce the remaining processed food I was consuming, and keep track of it all by writing about it in a daily journal—holding myself accountable.

So did it work? Mostly.

The most important lesson I learned, which may seem obvious, is that *I* control what *I* put into my body as well as the environment in which *I* consume my food. As soon as I made one change in eating habits, for better or worse, I noticed other changes immediately. Yet this wasn't always the case. I now start from a foundation of relatively clean eating, which means if my quality of sleep changes or if a chronic health problem such as allergies rears its head, it can most likely be traced back to how I fed my system in the proceeding days.

During my experiment for the book, the biggest change I made, which affected everything else I ate, was simply taking out the spoonful of sugar I put into my morning cup of coffee. This small change had a huge ripple effect. Without knowing it, this teaspoon of morning sugar was setting me up for poor eating habits the rest of my day. Now, I start my day without any sugar, and the crashes and cravings which plagued my day have disappeared.

So where should you start? Food information and education is being thrown at us from every angle and can be contradictory in nature. The USDA, the governing body that many people look to for unbiased health information, has multiple missions and partnerships in both the dairy and meat industries, categories of food that nutritionists encourage people to cut back on.[98] Instead of relying on someone else to tell you which particular foods are "good" or "bad," start to begin your changes with food in the way in which you socialize around eating, not necessarily in changing the food itself. Start by serving yourself meals on a smaller plate. Sit to eat with family or friends and mindfully enjoy your meal. If you finish what's on the smaller plate in front of you, wait a few minutes to digest and then see whether you're still hungry before you automatically reach for seconds.

Maybe for you, eating local food is most important. Join a CSA (community-supported agriculture, made up of local farms) to get fresh ingredients delivered to your door, which also cuts down on the stress of grocery shopping. If this is too much for you to take on yourself, see whether your company or coworkers are willing to get involved to either share a portion of the food delivery or have the company order their own portion so the cafeteria can start providing healthier, more sustainable options. You can even ask HR to start out with a simple no-cost change: rearrange the cafeteria buffet offerings so that the first 3 items in line are the healthiest. It's been shown that 66% of your plate gets filled up with these three items,[99] which means you can subconsciously start eating healthier today.

Bonus: If we retool our diet and our wellness habits to focus on health-promoting foods, we can actually reverse bodily damage[100] and repair it in such a way that medication taken to control chronic illnesses may no longer be necessary.

What if we looked at every piece of food we are about to eat and ask ourselves, "What will this do to my physical system? What will this do to my emotional system? Will I be happy if I eat this?" If we do all this work and still cannot significantly change the way we consume food, maybe something else is coming into play.

It's up to each person to sift through the information and experiment to see how what you eat makes you feel. I'm not saying you have to give up eating cheeseburgers, skip bacon at brunch, or swear off ice cream for the rest of your life. What I *am* saying is that you should be more conscious about where your food comes from and what ingredients make it up. This understanding will help you make smarter, more nutritious choices. I'm not going to lie: it takes time and effort and will not always be easy, but your choices will become habit, which then becomes a healthier lifestyle, which will definitely make you a happier person.

Easy Changes That Will Improve Your Food Future

Try these quick tips to change what you put in your body.

- Eat home-cooked meals more than you eat out.
- Put more vegetables on your plate than anything else.
- Preportion your food if you're going to eat in front of the TV.
- Buy smaller plates so you can start to eat smaller servings.
- Eat slower, giving your brain time to register when you're actually full.
- Read the labels on your food to make smarter buying decisions.
- Support a local CSA to get fresh local food, which often comes at a reduced price from what you'd spend at the grocery store.
- Sign up for a food subscription service that delivers healthy sustainable ingredients to take the planning and guesswork out of it for you.

INTERVIEW: How what we eat contributes to our overall health with Dr. Robin Berzin, founder of Parsley Health, a functional medicine practice based in New York City

There is a lot of talk in wellness circles about the search for "optimal health" through diet. What is optimal health?

Dr. Robin Berzin: Optimal health is a state where you feel energized, awake, and calm, where your weight is not destructive to your body, where you feel capable and enthusiastic about moving in some fashion every day, where you sweat 20 of 30 days a month and don't have evidence of inflammatory disorders from brain fog to acne to joint pain to colitis. If you're a female, you should be cycling regularly, not having severe PMS. A lot of people live day-to-day with stuff that isn't normal, but they just deal with it. You're not always going to feel 100% energized and 100% happy. Sometimes you will feel tired, down, or anxious, but is this something that comes and goes, or is it dominating your life? If you feel like there's something getting in the way of living to your fullest potential, then you want to look at that not as a thing to attack and destroy, but as something that is trying to tell you something about your body.

Can we achieve optimal health by the way we eat?

DRB: Absolutely. I have a chef who took gluten and dairy out of her diet, and her menstrual cycle, which had been gone for years, came back, her cystic acne went away, and her migraines went away. It's unbelievable how the foods we are eating are making us feel horrible on a day-to-day basis, but we are so habituated to eating a certain way and the people around us tell us to eat a certain way, but the norm doesn't always serve you. A lot of health issues can change by changing your diet.

When someone is suffering from chronic ill health, is it important to examine diet as a possible culprit?

DRB: Diet is the key to health. What you put in your mouth every day is determining the resilience of your body, how well your immune system works, what levels of information are present, and how well your cells are able to make energy or ATP (adenosine triphosphate), which is our energy currency. When I see somebody that has anything from digestive issues to auto-immune disease to anxiety, I always look at what they are eating because foods can cause any of these problems. A lot of people are eating inflammatory foods that don't work with their bodies very well and other people are sensitive to foods and don't realize it. When we can get underneath what people are eating and use food as medicine, people have much better success than if they just look for a pill.

Gut health seems to be on everyone's radar right now. What is gut health, and how does having a healthy gut impact our overall health?

DRB: Gut bacteria impact everything, from our thyroids to our brains to our personalities to how much fat we store. If you're feeding your bacteria the wrong foods or foods that are encouraging certain bacteria to live over others, those bacteria are going to influence your personality, your mood, and how much weight you gain. It's very interesting now to understand that we are a complex ecosystem influenced by our environment both internally and externally. New research on gut bacteria has been coming out every week for the last 5 years due to the Human Microbiome Project. Looking at the microbiome and understanding how one round of antibiotics can impact your microbiome for up to a year, how we've been on this crusade to destroy our bacteria and sanitize everything when we don't even understand the degree to which that is impacting our microbiome, how taking OTC drugs impacts your microbiome—there's so much we don't know. I think what we're uncovering now is how much we don't know about the role of bacteria.

Fifteen years ago, knowledge about celiac disease was not as widespread as it is today. Today gluten-free options are everywhere, and many people who do not have celiac are eating gluten-free diets. Is following a gluten-free diet beneficial or potentially harmful if you do not have a diagnosed gluten allergy?

DRB: Some people who go gluten-free reap benefits because effectively they are cutting out refined carbohydrates from their diet. Refined carbs are effectively sugar, which is extremely inflammatory and leads to everything from dementia to diabetes to hormone imbalances. Some people go gluten-free and benefit because they're not eating breads, cookies, cakes, or crackers anymore. Yet the preponderance of gluten-free products is problematic because some people think "oh it's gluten-free, so it's healthy," but basically they are eating a gluten-free version of the inflammatory foods. Having a gluten allergy and celiac disease is different than having a gluten sensitivity. What people find is if they are truly gluten-free for three weeks, which is how long it takes for your immune systems antibodies to reposition themselves, and then return to eating gluten, you're going to see the reactions to that gluten, if you're sensitive to it. If you cut it out and note how you feel, then reintroduce gluten and see changes in your skin, in joint and body pain, in digestion, even in mood, then you are probably reacting to the gluten. Gluten makes some people angry, as there are trans contaminants in the brain. If you have trans contaminants antibodies, you can form a reaction to gluten, which could be having profound inflammatory effects in the brain. A lot of people eat gluten and think, "I don't feel bloated, I must be fine," but it's not always a digestive issue that's at play. You really have to do the proper elimination and reintroduction to see whether you're allergic to gluten. Not everybody interacts with gluten the same way. You can also develop a gluten sensitivity at any point in life. Just because you were not sensitive 5 years ago doesn't mean that you're not sensitive now, and the only way to know is to do a proper elimination diet.

Paleo, pescatarian, flexitarian, vegan, macrobiotic—it seems giving yourself a dietary label in America is trendy these days. Do you recommend any one diet over another, or is the "everything in moderation" approach acceptable?

DRB: Everything in moderation is not a good idea, as we live in America where we're surrounded by really crap food that nobody should be ingesting. There is no one right diet for everyone. Some people do better on a more Paleo diet where they restrict carbohydrates, while others do better on a more low-fat vegetarian diet. The best cardiovascular research is on a Mediterranean diet, which has good healthy fats and lots of vegetables. The data is still out on Paleo and what that will do to your body long-term on a cardiovascular level. Dairy can be very inflammatory. Number one should be the quality of your ingredients: is it pasture-raised beef, is it organic non-GMO foods? The role of GMO is playing out. We don't yet truly understand whether GMO is good or bad; we've been genetically modifying food for thousands of years through cross-breeding or gene insertion and don't fully understand the impact of this on the environment or on human health, which is why it should be at minimum labeled. But the quality of your ingredients—whole ingredients, not refined grains but whole grains, low sugar—these are things you can't argue with. If you cut out processed foods, cut out sugar, eat whole organic, pasture-raised, free-range food, this will solve 80–90% of most people's problems. Within the remaining percentage, some people depending on genetics, environment, and stress levels, they're going to benefit from a different kind of diet, but that's something where people have to be really willing to live their way to the answer. Cut out the toxicity and then perfect the balance of micro-/macronutrients for you.

I'm on the road for half of the year outside the United States and am able to maintain a healthy lifestyle when I travel. I tend to lose weight on the road, and my diet is made up of fresh local food. When I return to the United States, I often put on 5 pounds. I'm convinced this is because of sugar. Is there science behind my theory?

DRB: Sugar is a big culprit for weight gain, but so is not moving enough. Sitting behind a desk all day is a big culprit with weight gain and stress is a big culprit with weight gain. The second you travel from your home base, you're not snacking as much or food isn't as readily available—you have to specifically go get food in a different way. You're also moving and running around—ultimately, you're less stressed out, and high cortisol levels lead to weight gain and inflammation. It's the relaxation that allows the body to let go of the weight. So many people when they travel live on restaurant food and eating at airports—eating much worse than they eat at home and feeling much more stressed out and sleep-deprived. It really depends on how you choose to travel. Yet all in all, refined sugar (agave, brown, white, liquid, etc.) and sugar mimickers are toxic, and it is incredibly important to get it out of your diet.

The idea that food affects your mood and can impact behavior was first introduced in 1973 by allergist Benjamin Feingold. What have we learned about the validity of this concept? In your own practice, have you seen examples of this?

DRB: Food affects moods and behavior through a couple of mechanisms. If you're sensitive to a food and that food is causing inflammation, the chronic turning on of your immune system, that inflammation affects the brain. Just this year, scientists proved that the lymphatic system, which carries your immune cells, extends through the dura (a thick membrane around the brain) into the brain. Historically, we always thought the brain was sealed off somehow from the immune system. Now it's very clear that whatever is happening in terms of inflammation and immune activity in your body is also happening in your head. This is affecting what neurotransmitters are made and how your brain and nervous system are working. People who are deficient in magnesium oftentimes have a lot of anxiety or hyperactivity in their nervous system. A lot of people who are stressed leech magnesium out of their systems faster, meaning sometimes a bad mood may be a nutrient deficiency. Low mood and low energy could also be a lack of B vitamins. Many people are deficient in B vitamins or activated B vitamins, called methylated B vitamins, because, genetically, people need methylated versions to use them properly.

Tell us a little about vitamins and supplements. If you eat a balanced diet of whole foods, do you need to take vitamins and minerals in pill form?

DRB: I use vitamins and supplements in a very targeted and strategic manner to achieve certain goals. The supplements I use are typically around a gut healing program to lower inflammation, working with the nervous system or hormone system, all based on testing and knowing a patient really well. It's not about just plying people with random supplements and taking them forever, as I don't think most people need most supplements forever. Now, that said, for most people living a busy modern life, there tend to be things that they really benefit from on an ongoing basis because they are not getting them in their diet and because the bodily demand and stress that they are under in day-to-day life means they have higher requirements. B vitamins, especially methylated folic acid, and methylated B12, probiotics—because a lot of people find their digestion is better. We're living in sterile environments, and from an immune perspective, a lot of people do really well when they have a probiotic regularly. It's not a one-size-fits-all solution, I don't believe in that. I do find that most people do better with B12 and probiotics and vitamin D, because people tend to be really low on it and not realize it, and that is important for musculoskeletal health and for immune health and inflammation. I also look at magnesium a lot, as many people do better with magnesium glycinate or ionized magnesium on a daily basis because it helps you sleep and helps calm your nervous system, and we're low on it because of stress levels. Antioxidant balance is also huge. If you are on the go, eating restaurant food and not a lot of high-variety fresh whole vegetables, then you should be taking a phytonutrient supplement that has all of the antioxidants that come from eating a big array of brightly colored vegetables because all of those phytonutrients are cofactors and they are important for making energy. Making sure you're getting good fatty acids is important: olive oil, coconut oil, and organic sunflower seed oil. Omega-3s from flax, walnuts, other seeds; some people do better with a fish oil supplement because they are not getting enough in their daily diet for their body. That's where it becomes a personal thing. These are things I see people chronically not having enough, and they feel better when they get them.

When I talk to people from other countries that visit the United States, almost all of them comment on the portion sizes served in restaurants. In a word: huge. How has this contributed to our eating issues in the United States, and would eating smaller portions correct any of our health issues?

DRB: Everyone should learn to chew more slowly and learn to eat to the degree that they're full. It all depends on the person; some people are really depleted and need to eat more, while others are chronically overeating. We are not meant to have mass caloric abundance constantly available. Our bodies are not designed to be constantly eating. We have an energy input overflow metabolically that causes damage to the body, which causes energy storage and weight gain. Expectations around portion size are problematic; learning to eat until you're full is an issue. People chronically overeat carbs and fried foods and stuff that is an energy glut to the body, and that causes metabolic disarray. I would love for people to eat smaller portions—get a meal and share it. You don't have to live on rabbit food, but if you are going to eat other foods, you need to not overeat. We have a culture that massages emotional distress with food. Food is cheap, widely available, and a low-effort way to make yourself feel energized, awake, and happy. But what about meditation, rock climbing, yoga, or running? These are ways to feel energized, awake, and happy that aren't destructive, something that no one teaches us at a young age. What can you do for yourself to feel better that doesn't involve food?

7

LIVING WELL
ON THE ROAD

"Ok, I just need another hour of sleep and I'll feel better," I tell myself as I swallow two more Excedrin with a swill of Diet Coke in my empty hotel room. I lie down and pull the covers back over my head to block out the light seeping through the sides of the window shades. A pulsating migraine has taken hold, and I'm nauseous from the pain.

An hour later my alarm rings again, and I drag myself out of bed, throw on leggings and a t-shirt, splash water on my face, and race downstairs to the parking garage, hoping I can make it to Sea-Tac airport in Seattle without missing my flight. I'm cutting it extremely close and praying that my airline status allows me a little leeway. Pulling up to curbside check-in, the sky cap glances at me in a way that tells me it looks and smells like I've been on a bender, when in reality this is what stressed out, burned out, overworked me looks like.

I tip him to take my bag and sprint toward security, while at the same time calling the rental car company to let them know that their car is sitting at the departure terminal. I hear my name over the loudspeaker for final boarding at the gate as I hand over my ticket, breathing hard and feeling ready to puke. Scrambling down the aisle, I take my middle seat and promptly pass out for the 5-hour flight. When I finally make it home to my bed I'm feeling a bit better, but know that I'll be calling in sick tomorrow. If there was ever a time to use a sick day, it's now.

CHAPTER 7

I would like to tell you this was the tipping point for me, that Aha! moment where things clicked into place and forced a dramatic change in the way I was living and traveling, but I'd be lying if I did. In reality, progress is slow, especially if you don't know what steps you need to take in order to meet your end goal. All I knew in this moment was that I was exhausted and I didn't have the brain or body power to do anything except lie still and hope I could figure out what to do next—after I got some much needed rest.

As my work travel schedule wasn't about to let up anytime soon (and I truly did love being on the road), the next few years became about focusing on what I needed to do to stay healthy both when I was at home and in some foreign place outside of my normal routine. Some of these steps you've already read about. I started to cook more and eat out less, leave work, and head to a yoga class instead of meeting my friends out for a night on the town, or grab a book and bike up the West Side Highway looking for the perfect spot in the sun instead of sitting motionless in front of the TV on Saturday afternoons. Once I was able to parse the "feel-good" from the "not-so-feel-good," I established a routine at home that made me feel so much better. Only then was I able to carve out time during my work trips to replicate these moments that kept me grounded, happy, and healthy and in turn made me better at my job.

When traveling to Los Angeles, I started to book my hotel stays near the beach in Santa Monica so I could take advantage of the time difference and go for a run near the water before I started my day. In Vegas, I researched restaurants for company dinners until I found one that was farm-to-table yet met the needs of the clients we were entertaining. After a crazy week of meetings in Florence that culminated in a runway show and party, I slipped out before the last round of drinks and strolled back to my hotel, taking in the beauty of the city at night and having a Zen moment all to myself.

Travel was part of my job, a part of my job that I loved. It's encoded in my DNA and it led me to seek out career experiences where I could use travel to my advantage. The moments of wellness that I learned to cultivate over the years began contributing to my wellness on the road in a big way. Travel gives

Get Well: In the Hotel

- **REST**: Sleep naked. Turn the temperature down to 65°, the optimal sleeping temperature, and let your skin breathe.
- **FIT**: Use the desk or chair back like a ballet bar for leg lifts or pushups to get your energy flowing in the morning.
- **ZEN**: Before you get out of bed every morning, sit up and do a 5-minute meditation to set the tone for your day.
- **LOCAL**: Make a reservation at a boutique hotel that has charm and character so you don't forget what city you've landed in this time.
- **FOOD**: Call ahead and ask for the minibar to be cleared out. This way you're not tempted by high sugar, high salt junk food. Instead, stop at a local grocery store and pick up your own goodies.

you a new perspective on life. Travel disrupts your habitual brain pathways and allows you to learn from what is happening around you. Travel affected my personality by allowing me to be more open, more creative, and more conscientious. Travel allowed me to be better at my job and at my life.

BEAM ME UP, SCOTTY

> *Travel is fatal to prejudice, bigotry, and narrow-mindedness.*[1]
>
> —Mark Twain

Business travel is essential for many companies and represents a substantial segment of the U.S. economy. In 2012, U.S. businesses spent $225 billion on domestic travel, which supported 3.7 million jobs and generated $35 billion in taxes.[2] Favorable market conditions typically lead to an uptick in business travel, but interestingly, historic data from 2007 to 2011 showed that businesses in 61 sectors of the market spent the most on business travel through our biggest recession in recent history, which in turn led to higher growth in profits following these years.[3]

People who travel for a living see the benefits in face-to-face meetings, especially during economic downturns. Taking time to meet a prospective customer in person, showing that you and your company are willing to go the extra mile even in hard times, makes clients feel at ease. These prospects are twice as likely[4] to become customers due to in-person meetings, and account managers believe that 42% of these customers would eventually be lost[5] if in-person meetings were to fall by the wayside.

The Global Business Travel Association (GBTA) estimates that future U.S. business travel spending will grow 3.2% in 2016 and 3.5% in 2017, reaching $299.9 billion and $310.4 billion respectively.[6] This is a wonderful steady increase and an area that businesses should consider allocating more resources to, especially since detailed statistical modeling looked at over an 18-year period across 14 industries indicates that for every dollar invested in business travel, U.S. companies have experienced a $9.50 return in revenue.[7] And it's not just the United States that is benefiting from business travel. Companies around the globe, especially those in emerging markets such as China, India, and Brazil, are contributing to the growth of global GDP, which has allowed business travel spending to rise worldwide to $1.1 trillion.[8]

Some people love to travel for work. It's in their bones. They feel at home and more like themselves when on the road than anywhere else. I know because this is how I feel. One in 4 business travelers say they get their best ideas when traveling, and 9 out of 10 mix pleasure into every business trip.[9] Many people who have built a career around travel actually enjoy spending time at the airport and can even use the time at 35,000 feet to network. The lines between work and life have already become blurred, but when you're on the road it's even harder to separate, as your free time can become unpaid work time if you're not careful.

According to a 2011 Columbia University study, all this travel can be *really* bad for our bodies.[10] Travelers who spend too much time on the road show signs of obesity, lack of sleep, and too much sitting, all of which takes a toll on overall health and well-being.

How Business Travel Is Changing

"Evolve or die" is a popular refrain among businesses. Here's how the face of business travel is changing, and if companies want to stay competitive, they need to pay attention.

- 32% of business travelers younger than 30 book their trips via smartphone.[1]
- Millennials are four times more likely to pay for onboard WiFi when in the air.[2]
- People announce their positive and negative travel experiences through social media.
- Travelers are extending their trips over the weekends in order to tack on leisure time.
- 54% of business travelers bring family members with them.[3]

NOTES

1. O'Brien, James, "Understanding the Digital Habits of Millennial Business Travelers," *Skift*, November 2014.
2. O'Brien, James, "Understanding the Digital Habits of Millennial Business Travelers," *Skift*, November 2014.
3. Peltier, Dan, "Business Travelers Unsure If 'Bleisure' Travel Is Allowed, but Doing It Anyway," *Skift*, October 22, 2014. https://skift.com/2014/10/22/business-travelers-unsure-if-bleisure-travel-is-allowed-but-doing-it-anyway/

This is why today's savvy business travelers have learned to create a hybrid experience, cultivating their own way of travel that carefully weaves together business and leisure. In 2013, a survey of business travel managers said that health and wellness was a mega-trend that would affect how their employees travel for years to come.[11] "Our research shows that there is a new mindset in today's business traveler," said Chris Rossi, a spokesperson for Virgin Atlantic. "They're not just a business person on their way to a meeting, but an individual thinking about making the most of every opportunity they find themselves in."[12]

Companies are starting to take a step back and realize that if they want their employees to stay happy and healthy on the road, they are going to have to adapt to the quickly changing needs of the travel environment. Airbnb recently expanded their business travel program making it easier for companies such as Google, SoundCloud, and TBWA\CHIAT\DAY to use their services for business trips. Goldman Sachs and Salesforce started allowing their employees to use Uber over car services, accounting for the company's 417% growth of ground transport in business expenses in the last year.[13] And a new company called Suitebreak is working behind the scenes with corporations to incentivize employees to bank wellness dollars and use them toward travel experiences.

It's not just Fortune 500 companies that are expanding offerings in order to make travel easier and healthier; airports and hotels are getting into the act, too. Health conscious and farm-to-table restaurants have been popping up around the globe and at airport terminals near you. At Logan in Boston you can find Berkshire Farms Market in Terminal B, which sells local made-to-order smoothies and sandwiches. SFO in San Francisco features Napa Farms, and LAX in Los Angeles led the charge when it introduced vegan favorite Real Food Daily to Terminal 4 in 2012.

But it is JetBlue at JFK's Terminal 5 in New York City that has launched some of the most groundbreaking wellness travel ideas yet. In 2015, the company debuted a 24,000-square-foot "farm," where they are growing herbs and the blue potatoes used to make the Terra Blues potato chips that JetBlue offers year-round as complimentary snacks to passengers during flights.[14] Located curbside at the arrivals area, this urban garden uses 2,300 milk crates to create the raised-bed farm which supplies some of the terminal's restaurants, donates ingredients to local food pantries, and allows area students to visit and learn about urban farming.[15] And the innovation doesn't stop there. The soil used in the urban farm is actually created from the 300 pounds of food waste taken daily from Terminal 5, which is hauled upstate and composted.[16]

It's not all about healthy food on the road either. You don't need to leave your fitness behind when you head out of town. Yoga rooms have popped up in airports: at O'Hare in Chicago, Heathrow in London, and Kainuu in Helsinki. Equinox fitness clubs recently announced that in 2018, it would open its first

Use Food to Keep You Healthy on the Road

Gut health is essential to keeping your immune system in balance, and when you are constantly traveling, you're changing and challenging that balance in a number of ways. Commit to healthy food choices on the road to keep your gut flora robust and stave off excess weight gain with these simple tips:

- Pack an emergency snack pack of almonds, carrots, nut butter, etc., for the plane or if you get hungry at odd moments due to time changes.
- Stay away from the salad bars, as you never know if the offerings have been cleaned properly or how long they've been sitting there.
- At the airport, search for apples, hummus, raw veggies, tea, or nut butters. These nutrient-dense foods will fill you up in a healthy way.
- Tell waiters about allergies or food sensitivities before you order to avoid confusion.
- Do your research on restaurants before you arrive and have an idea of what their healthy options are.
- Refuse the bread basket, which will only make you bloated and hungry.
- Take probiotics and travel with activated charcoal to ward off illness and keep your stomach happy. Ann Louise Gittleman, who holds an MS in nutrition education from Columbia University, says, "Open up an activated charcoal capsule and sprinkle on foods that are raw, undercooked or otherwise questionable. Charcoal is a wonderful all-around absorber of toxins and contaminants."[1] If all else fails and a food court is your only option, keep it simple and go for a salad, or rice and beans with some avocado to sneak in your healthy fats.

NOTE

1. Hyman, Mark, "10 Strategies to Eat Healthy While You Travel," June 26, 2015, http://drhyman.com/blog/2015/06/25/10-strategies-to-eat-healthy-while-you-travel/

hotel in New York City, where their branded building will feature indoor and outdoor pools as well as a 60,000-square foot gym. The company's goal is to reach 75 hotels worldwide.[17] Business travelers are rejoicing at all these new developments. "It's notoriously hard to stay healthy while traveling," say Alexia Brue and Melisse Gelula, founders of Well+Good. "But now hotels are making it easy to stay active with things like run concierges and sneaker-loaning programs. Hospitality brands now see their fitness and wellness offerings as what sets them apart from other brands."[18]

Business travel can be a solitary activity at times, with long periods alone between business meetings and plane rides with noise-canceling headphones, which essentially shut out the world. Getting out of your hotel room or resort to connect with people and with nature will help you to unwind, reduce stress, elevate your mood, and get you fully engaged in your surroundings. Even if the thought of it makes you uncomfortable, remember: life happens when you get outside your comfort zone. And it is this life experience that makes you better at your business.

Get Well: At a Trade Show

- **REST**: Change up your footwear. Women, try to find a cute pair of flats that will get you through the day.
- **FIT**: Alternate between sitting and standing throughout the day. You burn more calories when standing.
- **ZEN**: Every morning before you open your booth or walk the floor, stop, close your eyes, and take 5 deep breaths, sending positive thoughts into the space ahead of you.
- **LOCAL**: Take a "smoke break" and use 10 minutes to walk outside (away from the florescent lights and any real smokers) to feel the sunshine.
- **FOOD**: Hit the grocery store so you can pack your lunch. If you choose wisely, the prepared food section offers more nutritional value than anything you'll get from a trade show buffet line.

FIGHT FOR YOUR RIGHT

> *The act of traveling has yet to be seen as an essential part of our lives.*[19]
>
> —U.S. Travel Association

The United States has earned the nickname "No Vacation Nation." By law, those who hold jobs and pay taxes have no access to minimum paid leave requirements. In today's uncertain job market, the American workforce chooses not take time off because of fear of losing their job or the idea that their boss will think less of them. Many of us have even gone to work sick just to prove how dedicated we are. In Japan, the word karōshi means death from overwork, and while this might seem extreme, Americans are on a collision course toward burnout and even more serious long-term health problems, since we don't know how to take a timeout and focus on our self-care.

Just like we've developed nature deficit disorder, author William D. Chalmers says that U.S. workers are not taking the proper time off in effect creating a "Vacation Deficit Disorder." "America's Vacation Deficit Disorder derives out of a type of collective manic obsessive-compulsive disorder. One that has most Americans working longer and longer hours without the healthy physical and psychological benefits connected with taking vacations from their hyper-paced twenty-first century 24/7 electronic work leash."[20] In order to renew our well-being, we need to dedicate some hours to sleep, enjoy daytime rest, find ways to disconnect from work, and be able to get distance and perspective from our problems. The only way to effectively do this is by taking take a true vacation.

According to a 2015 *Skift* survey on American travel habits, 63% of Americans did not travel in the previous 12 months, and 42% did not take one vacation day.[21] True: when job security is nonexistent and the economy is unstable, the idea of travel seems like a luxury. Yet in the past year, 500 million vacation days went unused, leaving 53% of Americans feeling vacation deprived.[22] It seems like the answer is staring many of us right in the face. If you want to boost your happiness, strengthen

Employers Who Prioritize Time Off

U.S. companies are now realizing the benefits of having well-rested, less-stressed employees and are starting to put innovative vacation policies on the books. Here's a look at some current programs in place:[1]

Evernote—Withholds $1,000 bonus from people who don't take a minimum 1-week vacation.[2]

Full Contact—A $7,500 stipend is paid out yearly for a totally off-the-grid vacation.

HubSpot—Offers unlimited vacation days, plus mandatory 2 weeks off each year.

Netflix—Offers unlimited vacation days.

Rand Corporation—Provides 3% of monthly base salary plus regular pay for each vacation day taken. If all 20 days are taken during the year, employees receive an additional 5% of their annual salary.

TED—A 2-week office-wide summer shutdown happens where phones and email servers are turned off until everyone returns.

NOTES

1. Project: Time Off, "The Hidden Costs of Unused Leave," Oxford Economics Study, 2015.
2. Milligan, Susan, "The Limits of Unlimited Vacation," *Society for Human Resources Management* 60, 2 (March 2015).

relationships, increase creativity, and increase life satisfaction, then taking a vacation is absolutely nonnegotiable.

As early as 1962, author and historian Daniel J. Boorstin argued that people generally live alienated, inauthentic lives, and that during their holiday trip, they strive to escape to a more satisfying life.[23] In 2014, Americans spent $644.9 billion going after that authentic life.[24] We are a nation of consumption. Buying material goods and keeping up with the Joneses is a notion that is woven into the fabric of American life. Yet from your own personal experience, you know that we quickly adapt to these materials goods and soon are consuming more and more in order to replicate the initial rush. When *Time Magazine* published an article in 2011 on happiness, it asked people to think back to what brought them the most joy in the past 5 years. The report showed that experience, not material possessions, was the source of enduring satisfaction because experience shapes people into what they are today.[25]

Taking time out for vacation strengthens social and family bonds improving all of our relationships. Kids feel closer to their parents, when parents are able to detach from work and dedicate themselves to quality family time. A 2015 *Project: Time Off* study asked kids about their best memory of their parent in recent years; 61% of the answers had to do with a memory created while on vacation.[26] We have cultivated the next generation to understand that work is a priority, and these days it's become harder and harder to put down our devices and give 100% of our attention to any one thing. According to Lotte Bailyn, listening to the kids answers is the key, as there is "more time for good relationships to emerge under conditions that are not highly stressed."[27]

As a nation, we work to live, and now, over 50 years after Boorstin's observation, we are still having trouble taking time off to focus on family and self-care. At the end of 2015, Mark Zuckerberg, Facebook's founder, made headlines when he announced he would be taking a 2-month paternity leave to help raise his newborn. As a nation, the United States is so focused on work and defining our success by work that when someone, especially someone of Zuckerberg's stature, decides to put their family first or take some time off the grid to refresh themselves, it's looked down upon. This is not an issue in other developed nations. Australia has a mandatory 4 weeks off, the EU legally requires a minimum of 20 paid vacation days a year with some countries granting up to 30 days, and even though the Japanese are dying from overwork, at least they are trying to combat the problem by instituting 2 weeks of paid leave a year.[28]

Giving employees time off can actually benefit a company in a variety of ways. By letting employees take this much deserved time away, a company can determine whether they rely too heavily on one specific employee, identify opportunities for improvement, and create fail safes allowing for business to run smoother all around. The U.S. Federal Deposit Insurance Corporation (FDIC) has a long-standing position of encouraging banks to require a consecutive 2-week no-contact vacation policy to prevent embezzlement and fraud.[29] And according to the Society for Human Resources Management, employees who take most or all of their vacation time each year perform better, are more productive, and more satisfied in their jobs than those who leave time on the table.[30]

Yet U.S. workers who earn vacation time are only taking an average of 77% time earned off, roughly 16 vacation days a year.[31] These numbers are costing both employees and companies dearly. When you fail to take your vacation time, you are essentially working for free during days you've earned off, which leaves $65 billion in lost employee benefits[32] to go out the window every year. In 2015, the vacation liabilities held on the books by U.S. companies reached $224 billion.[33] These costs come due when a person retires or leaves a company and those unused vacation days need to be paid out. This is exactly why some companies institute a "use it or lose it" policy. People tend to view vacation days as a guilty pleasure, but companies should be touting the health benefits to employees and assessing the financial benefits for themselves.

When people are forced to take mandatory vacation or work up the courage to put in a time off request, it turns out 61% of these people are still working during vacation time anyway.[34] So why is it so hard for people to take time off? Do you feel you'll be seen as a slacker? Do you have too much to do? Are you worried everything will fall apart without you? If we understood the pitfalls of constantly working and being connected, would it make it easier for us to take a break?

Our environments and our habits influence our brain's neural pathways, which means they're also sensitive to change. New sounds, smells, language, tastes, sensations, and sights spark different synapses in the brain and may have the potential to revitalize the mind.[35] "When you go on vacation, your routine is interrupted," says Richard Branson, Virgin Group founder and

Take a Vacation; Create the Next Game Changing Company

According to the global consulting firm Sander Training, in a survey of 1,000 small business owners, one in five start-up ideas come to entrepreneurs while on vacation.[1] Here's a look at some of those brilliant ideas:

GoPro—While planning for his 5-month surf trip through the South Pacific, founder Nick Woodman came up with the action video camera.

Instagram—Founder Kevin Systrom was on the beach in Mexico when he remembered a photo class he took in Florence, sparking the idea for this photo-sharing app.

Lyft—CEO Logan Green had his Aha! moment for the ride-share service while he was on vacation in Zimbabwe.

Pravassa—In an outdoor restaurant overlooking the Red Sea in Egypt, the seeds of my wellness travel company were planted.

NOTE

1. Project: Time Off, "The Hidden Costs of Unused Leave," Oxford Economics Study, 2015.

one of the most successful entrepreneurs today. "The places you go and the new people you meet can inspire you in unexpected ways. As an entrepreneur or business leader, if you didn't come back from your vacation with some ideas about how to shake things up, it's time to consider making some changes."[36]

The effect of vacation on our cognitive flexibility along with its ability to shift focus and thinking reveals itself in many different ways. Out of our comfort zone in a new situation, we find creative ways to problem-solve, especially when we can't communicate using language. Research has found that when spending time in another country and culture, our creative output increases,[37] as we see how others live and how their approach to daily life and problem solving differs from what we're used to.

Real vacations, where you're able to mentally and emotionally detach from work, alleviate stress and burnout.[38] On vacation, we tend to spend more time outdoors or partaking in activities we don't get to do during our regular day. Some people seek out educational or learning vacations that allow them to engage their minds and bodies in a different way, saying goodbye to being sedentary at least for a short amount of time. In the past few years, 7.1 million adults have learned a new sport on vacation, while 6.6 million have learned a new skill such as cooking, photography, or dance.[39] When we really slow down and take time out for recovery to participate in active relaxation activities such as walking in the woods or going for a leisurely swim, it positively affects our sleep cycle not only during the vacation itself, but in the 2 weeks following our return home.[40]

Vacation is also good for our insides. Working overtime leads to ill health and commits us to an unhealthy lifestyle, if for no other reason than that we exercise less and eat fewer fruit and vegetables.[41] The Framingham Heart Study showed that middle-aged men who do not take vacation for several years are 30% more likely to have a heart attack.[42] And those men who changed their behaviors and decided to take more frequent annual vacations reduced their risk for mortality attributed to heart disease.[43] Women who step back from the job and go on vacation are more satisfied with their marriages,[44] and everyone who gets excited about their impending vacation increases their positive emotions and happiness.[45] While a vacation of 7 or more days is preferred, a weekend getaway can positively affect some areas of your health too: blood pressure, heart rate, and stress decline on a holiday after only 1 or 2 days.[46]

Throughout my corporate job experience, most of my bosses did not take vacation. They wore this as a badge of honor and commitment, and it sent a subtle message to anyone that worked for them that, effectively, employee earned vacation time wasn't important either. In reality, everyone needs time off to detach and recover, especially if you want to push yourself to do more or be better. This was revealed to be true when a study published in the *National Travel Leisure Monitor* showed that travelers experience a 25% increase in performance on vigilance tests after returning from vacation, and travelers 45 or older show a 50% increase in performance.[47]

Why You Should Be Paying Extra for the Airport Lounge

Not all airport lounges are created equal, but doing your research or joining a program such as Priority Pass, which operates in 160 countries and offers membership plans for every budget regardless of your airline status, may just save your health and sanity when it comes to frequent airline travel. Here's why:

- Lounges often have access to healthier snacks.
- The option to refresh by showering during a long layover may be worth the entry fee alone.
- There's no better place to sit when you have a flight delay, as free WiFi and workstations will allow you to be productive.
- Airport staff in the lounges are often senior agents who can rebook you, change your seats, or provide you with an upgrade if available.
- Instead of trying to find a cheap airport hotel to grab a few hours of sleep during an overnight, some lounges offer sleeping rooms or at least large comfortable couches so you can kick back and get some ZZZs.

When you travel, whether for business or pleasure, you have to adapt to practices that often take you out of your comfort zone. We've all heard the saying, "Life happens outside your comfort zone." According to psychologist Julia Zimmermann, the more one travels and engages in the practice of getting outside your norm, the more open you become and the more perspective you gain on life.[48] While the HR departments in some major companies may advocate for time off, pointing to high morale, company retention, and improved productivity as major reasons to book a getaway, it's time for each of us to realize that making vacation a priority makes us better workers and better people and improves every aspect of our lives. All of these things make you more valuable in any work setting.

CHAPTER 7

I WEAR MY SUNGLASSES AT NIGHT

Jet lag is for amateurs.[49]

—Dick Clark

We've all been there. Being awakened in the back of a taxi by a driver who's dropping you off at your hotel, downing your fifth cup of coffee at 11am just to stay alert in a meeting, or crawling into bed at 8pm for an entire week because you just can't keep your eyes open anymore. Welcome to jet lag. It sucks, and unfortunately it gets harder and harder to manage as we age or if we are frequently crisscrossing time zones. Sudden switches to the body's natural rhythms, such as having mood swings or not being able to concentrate, coupled with additional symptoms such as feeling sick, are what jet lag has in store for you.

Jet lag—a temporary issue affecting your body's circadian rhythm after crossing multiple time zones.

In 1883, standard time zones were created after long-distance train travel became popular. When jet travel became affordable in the late 1950s, a new problem arose; people were traveling longer distances across more time zones. The term jet lag, to explain all these symptoms, entered into popular lexicon after it appeared in the *Los Angeles Times* in 1966.[50] While jet lag is not preventable, it is manageable, and there are ways to cut down and even shorten the effects.

The body's biological clock sets your circadian rhythm, which regulates us to night, where the body temperature drops and melatonin production rises, and day, where the opposite affects occur. When traveling–between time zones, the body needs to experience outward environmental factors in order to reset its rhythmic patterns. The direction in which you're traveling also has something to do with it. Traveling east, ahead in the time zones, has been shown to have greater jet lag effects because our bodies are awake when it's actually time to sleep in your new destination. According to Smith L. Johnston, chief of the fatigue management team at NASA, it takes about a day to shift one time zone.[51]

Beat Jet Lag for Work

We've all been expected to take a red-eye and roll straight into a meeting. Saving time and money are usually the reasons behind this strategy for businesses, but the actual cost to a company can be a lot higher if you show up but cannot pay attention. Instead use these tips to combat the symptoms:

- **Arrive early**—Give yourself time to adjust to your new destination by arriving a day early. If that's not possible, then schedule your first meetings for the late afternoon so you have time to shower and take a nap.
- **Work your pretravel routine**—Once you find a routine that works for you (see my tips in this chapter), stick to it and you'll cut back on the dramatic jet lag effects you've felt in the past.
- **Control your light exposure** Catch the sunrise in the morning or sunset in the evening if you decide to adjust. Wear sunglasses on the plane or at anytime you want to diminish blue light to stay on your "home" schedule. Either path you choose, dimming hotel room lights and putting away any devices at least 1 hour before bed will help.
- **Stay hydrated**—Avoid alcohol and coffee 12 hours before you depart and drink only water on the plane.
- **Reset your clocks**—Watches, phones, computers, and any devices that you have should be set to your arrival destination when boarding the plane. This will help you mentally prepare for arrival.
- **Carry on**—Not having to wait for your luggage to arrive on the other end means you can head straight to your hotel and get started in your new time zone.
- **Reset your stomach**—Whether you choose to fast or not, you can reset your stomach by eating at regular mealtimes upon arrival. Focus on protein-rich breakfasts and light dinners so your body works during the day and can rest when it's bedtime.

- **Take melatonin**—Occasional short-term use of melatonin in pill form taken close to bedtime will help you deal with the changing time zones, reducing and in some cases even staving off jet lag.[1]

NOTE

1. Herxheimer, A., "Melatonin for the Prevention and Treatment of Jet Lag," *Cochrane Database Systematic Review* 2 (2002): CD001520. http://www.ncbi.nlm.nih.gov/pubmed/12076414

Want to make the change faster? The most effective way to do this is to use light. Our eyes process short-wave blue light via the melanopsin in the retina,[52] which signals our brains to stop melatonin production and stay awake. Scheduling this light exposure using both natural and artificial light helps to shift the body clock into the new time zone, but that's not all it will take. A study led by Harvard University Medical School professor of neurology Clifford Saper discovered that resetting your stomach might be a way to overcome the effects of jet lag.

Saper and his team found that fasting for half a day could help your body adjust to a new time zone.[53] If you are able to fast for an entire flight and then eat at the next normal mealtime in the new time zone upon landing, your body will adjust more quickly to the new schedule. This is how I have traveled for years, and I have found it one of the most effective ways to reduce jet lag or stave it off entirely. Additionally, the Harvard team looked at their research and its effect on animals. They found if animals have access to food as it related to their "normal sleep cycles, they will shift most of their circadian rhythms to match the food availability."[54]

Some experts suggest that trying to adjust your body for jet lag on a short trip that crosses only a few time zones is not worth it, New York to Los Angeles, for example, as it takes longer to properly adjust your body than the length of time you'll end up spending in that destination. While finding ways to manage jet lag is highly personal and individualized to your current body chemistry, creating a routine that works can mean the difference between a productive trip and one that ends with you face-down in your dinner plate.

Get Well: On the Plane

- **REST**: Prebook a seat that will allow you to be the most comfortable and either sleep or rest during your flight.
- **FIT**: Walk the aisles or find a galley way without flight attendants and get your stretch on.
- **ZEN**: Practice mindful breathing by tuning out all the sounds around you and listen to your breath.
- **LOCAL**: Smile at your fellow passengers and offer to help put up their luggage if you see them struggling.
- **FOOD**: Skip it. If you haven't brought your own snacks, use the opportunity to fast and let your digestive system rest.

TRAVEL WELL

Travel and change of place impart new vigor to the mind.[55]

—Lucius Annaeus Seneca, Roman philosopher

In 2008, 60 people gathered outside Buenos Aires, Argentina, for a long weekend. Having flown in from around the world, it was most attendees' first time in the country, and it was important to expose the group to Argentine culture. Staying on a former horse farm turned boutique hotel, guests were treated to organic meals at the farm and in local restaurants, cultural tours throughout the city, yoga, a massage workshop, and, of course, tango dancing. Years later, some still look back on this experience as the best immersive, experiential, and relaxing vacation they have had in years, especially as the stress of planning this vacation was alleviated for them. This was my wedding, and it was all attendees' first wellness travel experience.

Today, wellness tourism is a $494 billion industry that is currently growing at a rate two times greater than that of overall tourism.[56] Having run a wellness travel company for the last 7 years, inspired by that time in Argentina, this statistic is not a surprise to me. Today, travelers around the world have proactively decided that they'd rather eat healthy, relax more, prevent disease, and reduce stress in their daily lives. And they are

How Not to Get Sick When Traveling

Crossing time zones, sitting on a place with sick passengers, and sacrificing sleep can all be surefire ways to get sick when you travel. Keeping your immune system healthy and balanced year round is the first step in staying well, but try these added tips to keep sickness at bay while on the road:

- **Sanitize your seat**—Plane or train or bus, individual seats are not cleaned that often or that carefully. Travel with individual sanitizing wet wipes (I like ones with lavender essential oil), and before you settle in, wipe down the armrests, tray tables, and window area.
- **Drink water**—And lots of it! You get dehydrated from air cabin pressure and if you're traveling to a warm climate. The body is made up of 60% water, which keeps your digestion, circulation, body temperature, and brain balanced. When these things get out of balance, your body reroutes its resources to focus on these areas and leaves the immune system vulnerable.
- **Move**—Stretch your body in any way that you can. Movement relieves stress and tension, makes you feel better, and keeps your weight in check, especially if you're sedentary most of the day.
- **Sleep**—This should be a priority if you're away from home and out of your normal routine, as it's a time for your body to rest and recover. Don't try and pack everything in if you're on vacation, or beg out of a late-night drink if you're on a business trip in favor of getting more shuteye.
- **Wash your hands**—Shaking hands and touching money are two ways foreign germs get transmitted directly onto your skin. Don't take any chances and wash your hands regularly.
- **Take probiotics**—Tossing your food routine out the window is never a good idea as it'll make you feel like crap, but trying new foods is part of the adventure of travel. Use probiotics to maintain your gut health throughout your travel time, as keeping your gut flora healthy can limit the ill effects of introducing new food to your system.

not willing to give up these things when they travel. Ninety-six percent of people who've taken a wellness vacation have said it positively impacted their lives.[57] So the question is: why would you want to travel any other way?

Although wellness tourism is a new niche within the global travel industry, the practice of wellness-focused travel itself is not new—health spas, spiritual retreats, and hot spring travel have been around for years. These mentions might call up images of ground breaking retreat centers like Esalen Institute, which was founded in Big Sur, California, in 1962 (where Don Draper had his big breakthrough at the end of Mad Men), famous for its hot spring and educational programming that has a slight hippy bent to it, or Canyon Ranch, the luxury health spa launched in the 1980s in Arizona that focused on weight loss. A wellness vacation can be any trip designed to center on your well-being with added adventures, healthy food, fitness, or even the goal to return better than when you left. Yet you don't need a focused wellness vacation to enjoy the benefits of wellness travel.

Across the country, from millennials to executives, people are searching for ways to stop sacrificing their health for their job. Hotels catering to business travelers and overworked executives have also decided to get into the game. The InterContinental Hotel Group has recently opened the first business hotel chain, EVENhotels, completely dedicated to the health and wellness of its business travelers, California health spa VeraVia launched a corporate vitality program promising to teach executives tools for effective stress management and prioritizing nutrition on a busy schedule, and with ROAM Fitness now building gyms and shower facilities into airports past security checkpoints, wellness travel will be accessible at every price point.

CRAFT YOUR PATH

The world is a great book, of which they that never stir from home read only a page.[58]

—John Wade, author

Now that you've dug in and uncovered your purpose for getting well, it's time to take your carefully crafted routine with you.

Adding this tool to your toolbox and continuing to nurture it so it works for you means it will soon become second nature instead of a chore or something you have to remember to do. You may actually find yourself stopping mid-wellness to smile knowingly at how far you've come. Your wellness routine will become so natural and empowering, leading to a better quality of life, that you'll wonder how you ever made it through the day without it before.

After years of practice, I've perfected a wellness travel routine that works for me and makes the entire process less disruptive on both ends of the flight, whether for business or vacation. Bonus: it helps to combat jet lag too! Take the pieces that make sense to you or find some new ways to craft your perfect path to travel wellness. This pretravel road map (based on an 8+ hour overnight flight across time zones) will help you get started. For other in-flight and arrival ideas, flip to the checklist section at the back of the book.

T-MINUS 24 HOURS: BE IN BED BY 10:30PM

Make an extra effort to wind down even earlier on pretravel days. If you are lucky enough to be able to sleep on an airplane, the quality of sleep you get while in the air is nowhere near as restful as sleeping in your own bed—sorry business class travelers, I'm talking to you too. Any restorative sleep you get onboard is typically interrupted by background noise, in-flight entertainment, and meal service. While these influences can be mitigated by noise-canceling headphones, a great eye mask, and telling your flight attendant ahead of time that you won't be eating, failing to get a good night's rest can lead to increased hunger and the desire to eat more sugary foods along with refined carbohydrates. By showing up for your flight well-rested, you will not further drain your sleep cycle. Your body, your mind, and your waistline will thank you for this one.

T-MINUS 16 HOURS: GET IN A GOOD SWEAT

Whether you enjoy jogging, a group fitness class, or yoga, it is important to move your body before sitting stationary for a long period of time. Exercise reduces stress, burns calories, and keeps our muscles from succumbing to adaptive shortening (when the

Get Well: In the Car

- **REST**: Clearly sleeping while driving is a recipe for disaster. Before you head out on the road, make sure you get a good full-night's sleep, so you're not lulled to sleep behind the wheel.
- **FIT**: Stop the car every hour and get out and stretch your legs.
- **ZEN**: Play a game where you use each exit marker as a chance to mindfully focus on the road and nothing else.
- **LOCAL**: Not in a rush? Set your GPS to take the back roads and explore the areas you typically fly by.
- **FOOD**: If you're on a long road trip, plan ahead and pack healthy snacks, as you'll never find what your body needs at the gas station.

muscle fibers shorten and our range of motion is decreased due to inactivity). Consider movement as medicine. Exercise targets our muscles and connective tissues, lubricating our joints and moving cellular waste through our lymphatic system,[39] and it can also help to reduce jet lag symptoms faster. Exercise smoothens the adjustment to a new time zone by helping to reset your circadian rhythm. By getting your heart pumping and working out your stressors before you fly, you'll find yourself more sedate and ready for rest and recovery mode in flight.

T-MINUS 14 HOURS: DRINK YOUR VEGGIES

As the American diet moves away from meat and potatoes and toward quinoa and kale, we're progressing into more healthful eating habits. Yet if you spend more than one of your mealtimes in flight, you are missing an opportunity for optimal nutrition. Today, drink your greens for breakfast, ensuring that you get at least half of the daily recommended servings at once. If you don't have time to make your own morning smoothie, find a dark leafy greens option, which calorie-for-calorie has the most concentrated source of nutrition. While full of amino acids and protein, not all juices are created equal; therefore it is important to find an option that is not just a juice, but also has the fiber, the whole fruit or vegetable, still in the drink. With juice bars opening on every corner from Miami to Seattle, it has never been easier to grab a juice to go. To make sure you are maximizing the nutrients and fiber as well as choosing a low-sugar option, you had better take a look at that label.

T-MINUS 11-13 HOURS: GET UP AND MOVE

Any way you can find to add movement throughout your day will balance out the hours of sitting in your plane seat. Movement releases endorphins, which helps to trigger the relaxation response when you most need it. So whether you decide to take the stairs at the office, walk around the block the long way to pick up your lunch, or park at the farthest spot away from the door when running any last-minute errands, you'll increase your health and improve your mood as a bonus.

T-MINUS 10 HOURS: LUNCH

While you might already be stressed out about work piling up while you are away, do your body and your mind a favor—step out to pick up a healthy lunch and eat it mindfully away from all your electronics. Enjoy a light well-prepared lunch of your favorite green salad with lean protein, or quinoa tossed with seasonal veggies; choose your add-ons with care, opting for crunchy legumes instead of bacon and a high-quality olive oil dressing for salads.

T-MINUS 5-9 HOURS: DRINK YOUR WEIGHT IN WATER

Aircraft cabins are low in humidity, which leads to dry skin, dry eyes, and dry mucus membranes in your nose. Dehydration can often exacerbate jet lag, and partaking in alcohol and coffee in flight is a total no-no as it only further parches your system. Start preparing your body by upping your H_2O intake preflight and then drinking water en-route. Keep a reusable water bottle within easy reach and continuously sip from it all day long. Having to get up to refill that bottle or use the restroom serves two purposes: it gets you moving and replenishes your system.

Water rule: 4 cups for every 5 hours in the air.[60]

T-MINUS 4 HOURS: EAT A NUTRIENT- AND PROTEIN-RICH DINNER

Pass on airplane food. Aside from some meals being prepared in unsanitary conditions,[61] the food is bland, full of sodium, and not all that nutritious—basically a lot of empty calories. Instead, make sure that the meals you consume preflight are nutrient-rich (packed with a high percentage of vitamins and minerals per calorie), protein-heavy, and full of fatty acids. This kind of meal keeps you full and satisfied; also, consuming omega-3 fatty acids will help to keep your skin from drying out onboard. Grilled fish and dark green vegetables with a side of olive-oiled avocado is my typical preflight meal. If you eat meat, a lean protein such as a small skinless chicken breast would be a good substitute. *Insider tip: Flight attendants pack their own food. This should tell you something!*

T-MINUS 3 HOURS: PACK SNACKS

Packing snacks high in protein and fiber will keep you sated until you reach your destination. Almond butter, which falls under the high protein and fiber category, is also high in calcium and iron. Pack a small container (less than 3 ounces) to spread on celery or seven-grain bread (and smile big when you walk through security). Cooked whole grain pasta is also a good option to bring on board. You can choose your own accoutrements such as grated cheese, olives, peas, or sautéed mushrooms. Pack them separately and combine when ready. On a return flight, you don't typically have the ability to make your snacks, so instead stock up on raw unsalted nuts or low-sodium trail mix and grab some fruits such as a banana or apple at the airport before takeoff.

T-MINUS 2 HOURS: GET READY FOR BED

If you are going to be on a plane for more than 8 hours, hop in the shower before leaving home. Be sure to slather on organic body oil when you're done to seal in moisture and make your skin feel soft and supple in preparation for plane dehydration (this

Get Well: In the Airport

- **REST**: If you don't have access to the airport lounges, buy it. Try a yearly service like Priority Pass or purchase entry for the day and access a more quiet, tranquil space that often comes with healthier snacks and a place to shower.
- **FIT**: Wear your sneakers when you fly so you can walk laps around the airport before you board.
- **ZEN**: Resolve to let it go and become a master of patience as you pass through airport security.
- **LOCAL**: If your airport offers a connection to nature such as JetBlue's Terminal 5 at JFK or Changi's Nature Trails in Singapore get outdoors and get grounded.
- **FOOD**: If you can't eat healthy before your arrival, look for fruits and vegetables for their high nutritional value and to stave off bloating.
- **BONUS**: If you take more than two round-trip flights a year, consider investing in Global Entry or the TSA Pre-Check program. For a small fee and a background check, these services let you skip the security lines, leave your shoes on and keep your luggage packed reducing your stress levels and often even allowing you to arrive 20 minutes later at the airport. This is the best wellness travel hack I've learned in years.

oil goes in my hair and on my face as well). Dress in comfortable yet chic clothes, like loose linen pants and a plush sweater or a cotton t-shirt, and grab a cashmere scarf that can double as a blanket. I never wear makeup to the airport, but if you can't stand the thought of this, you should hightail it to the airplane bathroom once on board. Wash your face using your travel size face wash and your skin will be happy throughout the flight.

T-MINUS 1 HOUR: ASK FOR TEA

My nightly bedtime routine does not involve a cup of tea unless it is a very cold winter night. Therefore, tea before flying helps me to settle into a different rhythm. Traveling with your own tea bags ensures that you will have the flavor and natural sedative effects that you need to wind down from a busy, stress-filled day. Chamomile and valerian are my go-tos, and they taste yummy without milk or sugar, both of which aggravate your mucous membrane and lead to further dehydration. If these flavors don't appeal to you by themselves, there are plenty of companies that make bedtime teas with complementing spices. Most coffee shops or flight attendants will be happy to offer you a cup of hot water.

BONUS TIPS

- Once you find a preflight routine that works for you, multiply it by two and hit the go button 48 hours before departure.
- If you're leaving the office for vacation, set up your away message to start sending 48 hours before your departure. This will leave you room to handle any last minute emergencies before you actually depart.

By consciously constructing a pretravel wellness routine, you will come to learn that, if nothing else, you will feel better, be less stressed, and be less affected by jet lag when you arrive at your destination. Trust me, I've been doing this for years (both for personal and for business travel) and have seen the results to prove it.

Today's wellness travel market encompasses business and leisure travel along with organic restaurants, fitness studios, national parks, airports, and hotels. Every day, more and more industries are getting into the act. I know everyone would like to be happier, healthier, and less overwhelmed in some area of life. With the rise in stress levels and an aging population who has raised the upcoming generation to be wellness-focused, finding ways to live well both on and off the road is a lifestyle change that is here to stay. The power to control your well-being, no matter where in the world you find yourself, now rests in your hands.

Tips from Wellness Road Warriors

These hardworking entrepreneurs all hit the road in support of their businesses. Here are some of their must-do's when it comes to living well on the road[1]:

Sadie Lincoln, founder of Barre3 Fitness—Aim for 8 hours of sleep when traveling to avoid getting sick.

Kristin Dahl, nutritionist and author of *The Art of Wellness*—Pack digestive enzymes to help break down strange food. A healthy gut keeps your immune system strong.

Andrew McCarthy, actor, director, and travel writer—Don't eat airplane food. Instead pack almond butter to snack on.

Alexandra Bonetti Perez, founder of The Bari Studio—Avoid coffee and sleep medication to conquer jet lag. Instead, opt for calming herbal tea before bed.

Ethan Zohn, *Survivor* winner and co-founder of Grassroot Soccer—Always wipe down the seats, headrest, and tray tables with an antibacterial wipe on the airplane.

Latham Thomas, author and founder of MamaGlow—Grab a salad at dinnertime. Carry a travel-sized pouch of hemp seeds, which will fortify any meal on the go.

Charlie Knoles, founder of The Veda Center—Fast when you fly and eat your first meal on arrival in accordance with the local mealtime to manage jet lag.

Jared Koch, creator of *The Clean Plates Guide*—Spend 15 minutes online before you hit the road to research restaurants that serve clean food. This way you know where you can eat without compromising your lifestyle.

Kimberly Hartman, creator and sustainable designer of JADEtribe—Work out and drink lots of lemon water the morning you depart. This will prepare you to sit for a long flight.

NOTE

1. Schaffer, Linden, "Pravassa's Well on the Road Interview Series." www.pravassa.com

8

GET RESULTS AND SUSTAIN SUCCESS

"I love that you call it a practice," said Laura as she passed the bowl of quinoa across the table. "It clearly shows that you have to work at it, and it will get easier as times goes on."

We were sitting at the table on a cool fall night in Vermont, enjoying dinner on a wellness weekend that I curated. Laura, a newbie to wellness, had traveled cross-country to join our group for a few days in hopes to gain an understanding of self-care. Since her arrival, she had gained some tools; now she was aiming to see how they figured into her life back home. That night as she uttered her observations across the table, she was talking about yoga, but she might as well have been talking about life.

It took me 15 years to get to that table. Eighteen months earlier, I had been sitting in midtown Manhattan in a drab office on the 6th floor, overlooking 5th Avenue, turning down a promotion at work. As my bosses sat shell-shocked and slack-jawed, questioning how anyone could turn down running a multi-million dollar business, I sat there numb, knowing not what I wanted, but knowing that I did not want to spend more time and energy devoted to something that I wasn't devoted to at all. Six months later, I quit. A year after that I was sitting with a full belly, happy heart, and huge smile on my face in Vermont, with people who had assembled to focus on their well-being and a newbie so self-reflective that in 48 hours she'd summed up what took me 15 years to master.

The time to invest in yourself is now—not 15 years down the road. It's the twenty-first century, and the human race has survived so much. The developed countries in which many of us live have found ways to extend longevity. As Nesse and Williams write in their book on evolutionary biology, "The major causes of death for people in developed nations have shifted from disaster (starvation, war) and disease (smallpox, malaria) to decay (heart disease, cancer)."[1] If you picked up this book, it is because you love yourself. If you picked up this book, it is because you want to become more responsible for your well-being. If you picked up this book, it is because you are ready to make some lasting life changes. If you've made it to the last chapter of this book, you are ready to start living well on the road.

I CAN'T GET NO

What makes life interesting, finding the balance between cigarettes and tofu.[2]

—Gwyneth Paltrow

Let's face it: everyone would like to be happier, healthier, and less overwhelmed in some area of their life. Yet success isn't possible without change. Which means you need to shake it up a little bit and carve out a new path toward your goals. The key is to make a gradual, sustainable shift that is manageable, one that sets you up to succeed. Start today. Start from within. Build a solid foundation, a base that is healthy, one that enables you to grow and thrive.

Twenty-four hours a day, our bodies offer us built in feedback. We get hungry, tired, and horny, but there are many more signals that our bodies offers that we ignore because we're not used to listening, or we push them aside because there are more important things to do. For example, it's normal in our society to reach for a painkiller if we have a headache or are experiencing muscle pain. Over time, this trains our body to ignore its warning signs, to tune out the signals that a headache is approaching. Instead, learning to trust our bodies again, not just on this front but on every front, will provide the tools needed to make smarter, healthier decisions.

Developing our intuition, a word derived from Latin which means "knowing without explanation,"[3] is something anyone can do with a little patience and compassion toward oneself. Often we know a lot more than we give ourselves credit for; we know when something is off within our body or if we find ourselves in a situation that is just not right. It's important to acknowledge that intuition exists and learn to use it as a tool instead of ignoring or second-guessing it.

Chronic stress dampens not only our intuition but also our health. From all the previous chapters you've read, scientific literature has made it clear that sustained stress alters our biology and creates physical illnesses such as heart disease, strokes, and diabetes. The food we reach for to quell this stress causes inflammation, and the chronic anxiety we feel leads to negative emotions, which also manifest in disease. Yet many of the health problems we suffer are not because of genetics, they are because of the coping mechanisms we've created. We've programmed ourselves to reach toward a salve that acts as a Band-Aid instead of a healing tool. The famous Zen Master Thich Nhat Hanh says, "The present moment is the only moment available to us and it is the door to all moments."[4]

Common stressors in America are concerns over unemployment, not being able to financially afford our lifestyles, and not feeling like you have a sense of purpose. All of these things, while valid, are roadblocks, providing resistance and reasons that prevent us from making a change. It is hard to focus and enact real change when we cannot move beyond our fears. Change requires a new way of thinking. It is now up to you to decide that you're ready to open up to new things. It is up to you to define your purpose. It is up to you to shape your expectations and find the tools that work to further your ability to live well on the road.

Change is painful; much like a growing pain, you will experience discomfort when it comes to doing something new. Change itself amplifies stress. Yet sticking with it, repeating your new patterns, is how you turn change into success. Psychiatrist Jeffrey Schwartz and management coach David Rock say,

Practice this "I AM" Mantra

A mantra, Sanskrit for "sacred utterance," is a word or series of words we repeat to help shift our subconscious patterns of negative thinking. Employing words and sounds to create positive thinking has been used for years across various cultures and religions in order to guide people toward self-awareness. Today mantras are used in everything, from meditation to treating PTSD. Start your day with a few rounds of this "I AM" mantra to set your focus and a positive foundation for the day.

Sit quietly and focus on your breath.
As you inhale, say or think: I AM
As you exhale, say or think your phrase for the day.
Know you can always come back to a few rounds of this mantra anytime throughout the day to refocus your attention.

I AM examples:

I am ENOUGH	I am LOVE	I am PASSION
I am BRAVE	I am FEARLESS	I am OPEN
I am CAPABLE	I am STRENGTH	I am WORTHY
I am BEAUTIFUL	I am HAPPINESS	I am STILLNESS

"Trying to change any hardwired habit requires a lot of effort and often leads to a feeling that many people find uncomfortable. So they do what they can to avoid change."[5]

I've been reminding you that life happens outside your comfort zone. When we try something new, the prefrontal cortex of our brain is activated, asking our working-memory to analyze and compare new information to the area of the brain that works when we go about a routine, familiar activity.[6] This requires a lot of energy and tires out the brain quickly, therefore defaulting to our habitual patterns become the easier, less stressful choice. Trying to change that routine behavior requires a lot of effort, as we're overriding the part of our brain that is trying to signal that something is not right.

Neuroscientist Edmund Rolls linked the neural firing, what happens in our brains when experiencing change, to fear. When we activate the prefrontal cortex in new situations, "error" signals are detected, which push people to become emotional and act impulsively.[7] Before you know it, we choose not to put ourselves in new, uncomfortable situations. However, over time as you are able to push past the resistance to make a change, the brain releases neurotransmitters, stabilizing the brain circuits and allowing for this change to become the new pattern, the dominant pathways.[8] The more you concentrate on your area of change, the higher the attention density.[9] Do this over and over, and thoughts and actions are no longer new; instead, they start to be accessed from the habitual part of the brain.

With so much internal activity happening surrounding change, you can understand why it's easier to make small, manageable shifts rather than one big all-encompassing switch. Our habits are so hard wired and change often feels uncomfortable, so it's easy to understand why excuses such as "there's not enough time to figure it all out," "I don't know where to start," and "I'm afraid of what I'll find if I being to look" are all points of resistance. Remember, it took years to develop the habits and lifestyle you have now. It's going to take time before the changes you make begin to feel routine. You'll have to expect resistance from yourself and from others, especially if the changes you want to make affect more than just yourself.

Lack of commitment is a huge change-killer. Prioritizing what is important in order to make room for change is key. For me, sleep and fitness are at the top of my list. If I don't sleep well, I don't have energy. If I don't work out, I don't sleep well. (Notice a cycle here?) I've learned I need to forgo a late night out if it cuts into my sleep, or that I need to get outside and find a way to move if my fitness level is suffering. I need to do these things in order to feel well, be productive, and stay sane. After 7 years of putting these things first, they are ingrained. They no longer feel like work; when my body starts to crave them, I listen. Change is never easy. You have to learn to let go of what you think things should look like and focus on what you want them to look like. Often the hardest changes to make come with the most rewarding outcomes.

How to Initiate at Work

Social scientist Arthur C. Brooks writes, "People generally have a 'bliss zone,' a window of creative work and responsibility to match their skills and passions."[1] If you feel you're not reaching that state at the place you spend most of your waking hours, then it's time to make some changes. Whether its initiating an overall shift in office culture or just in the way you go about your day, it's important to create a plan and set goals so you can benchmark results and evaluate success. Once a plan is in place, follow these steps to see your goals come to fruition:

1. Effectively communicate the plan and its steps to yourself and/or your team.
2. Understand it won't be easy, but create a support network by surrounding yourself with cheerleaders and/or make sure you cheer on your team.
3. Check progress frequently to see how far you've come.
4. Get constructive feedback: either from your support network or those in the midst of change with you.
5. Be prepared to alter your plan on the basis of the data you've already collected.

NOTE

1. Brooks, Arthur C., "Rising to Your Level of Misery at Work," *New York Times*, September 5, 2015.

IF YOU BUILD IT

> *If you don't know where you are going, you might end up someplace else.*[10]
>
> —Yogi Berra

The first time I felt successful as an entrepreneur had nothing to do the size of my bank account, the number of trips I was leading, or the fact that I was paying people to help carry out my goals. It was 3 years ago in a little village in Rajasthan, India. My guide and I had stopped to sit in the afternoon sun and chat. After hearing his story, he asked me mine. Peppering me with questions: What was I doing in India? Why was I traveling alone? What did I do for work? With awe and wonder, he listened to my journey and in the end told me how amazing it was. His daughters would never have the ability to build something like I did because of the caste system they were born into. In his world, making new opportunities for yourself wasn't something they were able to do, and instead, they had a path already laid out before them.

It took a total stranger to hold up a mirror to my life to show me how far I had come. And as great as this feeling of success was, it also saddened me as in that moment I realized how many huge milestones I had passed, each a success in their own right, which I had failed to celebrate. I had worked so long and so hard, pushing myself every day at something I love, but I was always looking ahead and not pausing to be present, even though I had cultivated the tools that would allow me to do just that.

As Leslie Perlow wrote in the *Harvard Business Review*, "We are successaholics, not workaholics."[11] Growing up, we receive praise for getting good grades or when we win sports matches. The feelings we experience in these situations begin to be associated with success. As adults, the most common place for us to find that same sense of achievement is in the workplace. We get rewarded with promotions, larger salaries, and even awards when we perform well, which can lead to more power, more authority, and definitely more responsibility. And while all these things might look like a success from the outside, it's possible that at some point we rise beyond what actually makes us happy, beyond that "bliss zone," which instead leads us to overwork, burn out, and question our life's purpose. We are not addicted to our work, to the late hours, and to always having to be available; we are addicted to the feelings of success we are trying to elicit from that work. What if each of us was able to redefine what success looks like in our lives?

Russell Simmons, yogi and cofounder of Def Jam, has been vocal on the wellness changes he's implemented into his life

A Look at the Blue Zones

In 2004, Italian Gianni Pes and Belgian demographer Michel Poulain published a study on the prevalence of the one-to-one female-to-male ratio in a mountain town on the island of Sardina.[1] The researchers, along with American Dan Buettner, had, for the past four years, been studying this geographic area where people lead measurably longer lives in good health. After circling the area on a map with a blue marker, it subsequently earned its designation as the world's first "Blue Zone." The research team became so fascinated with this region and its wellness habits that it started to explore the globe to see whether any other populations fit similar criteria that appeared in this first Blue Zone.

As recently as 2008, Buettner, Pes, and Poulain have identified five different Blue Zones: Sardinia, Italy; Okinawa, Japan; Nicoya, Costa Rica; Ikaria, Greece; and the Seventh-day Adventists community in Loma Linda, California.[2] During the course of their research into these populations, Buettner and his colleges found that "life expectancy is as much as 10 years greater. There was as much as a 1/6 the rate of cardiovascular disease and a 1/5 rate of the big cancers like colon and breast."[3] So what is the secret to these pockets of populations that are able to lead long healthy lives?

It all comes down to their wellness routines. Each of these five Blue Zones has a through-line of habits that directly contribute to their everyday well-being: family is considered a priority, each person participates in constant physical activity, a plant-based diet is consumed, there is no smoking, there is a high level of social engagement, and there is an overall low stress level.[4]

Buettner was so enamored with these lifestyle concepts and the quality of extended life they produce that a few years ago he teamed up with Healthways, a national healthcare company, to create The Blue Zone Project™. Buettner's project is a systemic community approach toward better well-being, where long-term evidence-backed policies created and followed by citizens, schools, employers, restaurants, grocery stores, and community leaders hope to improve the health and longevity of its residents.[5] It remains to be seen if these planned communities will produce longer-living happier residents, but emulating the core principles of a Blue Zone lifestyle doesn't sound so bad.

NOTES

1. Poulain, Michel, and Giovanni Mario Pes, "Identification of a Geographic Area Characterized by Extreme Longevity in the Sardinia Island: The Akea Study," *Experimental Gerontology* 39, 9 (September 2004): 1423–29.

2. Buettner, Dan, *The Blue Zones: Lessons for Living Longer from the People Who've Lived the Longest* (Washington, DC: National Geographic Society, 2008)

3. Baldauf, Sarah, "From 4 Long-Lived Cultures, 9 Tips for Longevity," *U.S. News & World Report*, March 25, 2008.

4. Buettner, Dan, *The Blue Zones: Lessons for Living Longer from the People Who've Lived the Longest* (Washington, DC: National Geographic Society, 2008).

5. Blue Zones, "Our Approach," https://www.bluezones.com/services/our-approach

saying, "I used to think anxiety and insomnia drove me to success, but it was the stillness that let me be good at anything. When you extend the seconds of stillness, that's when you're able to think and learn."[12] It takes years to reach that Aha! moment that changes everything. All the experience, including the triumphs and the failures, build up, ruminate, and incubate into a breakthrough where things seem to fall into place and your path opens up in front of you. After years of priding herself on little sleep, Arianna Huffington fell and hit her head in an episode of exhaustion. She now dedicates herself to the topic of well-being and just launched her new venture, Thrive Global, which aims to change the way we live and work through wellness improvement the workplace. Oprah Winfrey has had a lifelong struggle with her weight and believes she finally found the key to her success when she shifted her thoughts around her body: "Gone, for me, are the days of wanting to be thin to fit into anything other than my best body and best life."[13]

Success is an investment. Making any change is scary, and feelings of doubt, uncertainty, frustration, and fear are normal. Entrepreneur Michael Dell's wise advice during the 2003 commencement address at the University of Texas at Austin was, "Recognize that there will be failures, and acknowledge that there will be obstacles. But you will learn from your mistakes and the mistakes of others, for there is very little learning in success."[14]

The investments of time, emotions, sweat equity, changes to the way you think, and even financial obligations (boutique fitness workouts, anyone?) are all required to reach success. Creating a structure and being honest with yourself about what you can accomplish and in what kind of time frame will set you up for victory. Use your fears to find out where you're vulnerable and motivate yourself to move beyond them. Fears show you what you hold as important. Are you afraid of being successful? The idea of reaching success itself can be an obstacle. If you're subconsciously blocking yourself from meeting your goals and getting what you really want, you could be stuck in this pattern. Be kind to yourself and know it is OK to feel joy, happiness, accomplishment, and pride.

Throughout the years, your concept of success will change and morph as you age and as priorities shift. Remember, success is a journey with many milestones along the way, not one big end goal. No one will ever be all done, as once you reach what you thought was your big goal, there will be another one waiting. Don't get sucked into the rat race of success. Instead, find meaning and purpose in the kind of success you want to achieve. Identify the reasons why you want to achieve it. Acknowledge that you might fail. Everybody fails. In fact, this is how you learn. You cannot understand or appreciate success if you don't have failure to compare it to. You cannot rise and be proud of yourself unless you've experienced what you've had to overcome to get to where you are. It's time to stop making excuses and accept responsibility for where you are now and where you'd like to be. Learn from the mistakes you've made in the past and let it focus you on the future. Don't give up if you feel overwhelmed. Instead step back, reevaluate, and take on a smaller task, one that you know you can accomplish. And if all else fails, "fake it until you make it!"

The power of positive thinking, once an esoteric concept, has been shown to alter levels of happiness.[15] However, even more effective than thought, researchers at Harvard University have begun to study the effects of power poses, physical postures that cause individuals to feel more positive, in control, and optimistic. Research has shown that the psychological effects of power poses—standing firmly on the ground with an open chest, sitting upright with your feet grounded in a chair, spreading your arms wide open—all enhance the brain's executive function, reducing stress and anxiety and making you more confident, captivating, and enthusiastic.[16] Power posing can improve quality of speech and shows to those watching, via body language, that we know what we're doing. Even if you don't, your body generates high testosterone and low cortisol in these moments, leading to psychological reactions that enhance our belief in ourselves.[17]

A LITTLE HELP FROM MY FRIENDS

Success doesn't happen in a vacuum. You're only as good as the people you work with and the people you work for.[18]

—Casey Kasem

Learning to ask for help can be a humbling yet freeing experience. I have always been fiercely independent, and asking for help has never been easy. A few years ago, I was in Capri, Italy, with some travelers hiking down an unmarked mountainside. I was not wearing the proper footwear and kept slipping and sliding every few feet. At one point, the person in front of me turned around and said, "You don't like to ask for help, do you?" as she reached out her hand to guide me down. In that moment, my face flushed. I felt embarrassed that someone could see me so clearly and relieved that I wasn't in the journey alone.

We've all heard the saying "like attracts like." After decades of research, Dr. David McClelland published *Human Motivation* in 1987, a book that delves into the psychology of motivation. Dr. McClelland's research concluded that while you might have the best training and best intentions, if you surround yourself with a group of people who exhibit behaviors that derail your goals, you will not accomplish them.[19] As your ideas of success start to take shape, make sure you're creating a positive support system to help you reach your goals. Look for mentors who have walked similar paths in order to gain direction, to feel connected, and to feel validated, or find a group to join that is working toward the same goals. Having someone to celebrate your success with or cheer you on when it's tough will actually spur better results in the end.[20] From fitness motivating groups such as roadrunners to weight loss support groups to meditation clubs that meet weekly, encouragement can be found in all forms. No one can be 100% 100% of the time, but if you feel better today than you did yesterday, great! If not, then lean on your network for support and start fresh again in the morning.

If creating a real-life support system seems a bit intimidating or you don't know where to begin, turn toward technology to help you get started. Having an app or program that helps measure progress with real data points can push you to take action on your good intentions. Currently, the most popular form of achievement apps is activity trackers, which provide feedback on physical behaviors such as calorie burning and sleep quality. Yet there are many apps out there that play on our psychological motivation, too, and prompt behaviors such as time management or connect you with an online community that is working toward achieving similar goals.

Asking for help hasn't become more comfortable for me over the years, but I have learned to recognize when I need it and that I cannot do everything alone. Radical honesty with myself, putting myself out there and showing my vulnerability, has not only pushed me out of my comfort zone but also allowed me to be successful and stay sane. Deciding to choose healthy behaviors and investing in my needs has allowed me to live my road to wellness. And while there are always twists and turns along the way, when I feel I can't go it alone, someone has always been there to offer me that helping hand.

Try These Apps to Boost Your Wellness

Recommended by those in the wellness community, download these apps to keep you on target when reaching your wellness goals.

Coach.me—A built-in community to help you reach all your wellness goals, from fitness to personal growth to learning a new skill, you can share your success with a group or hire a personal coach to rally you on.

MotionX 24/7—Track your sleep cycle, the quality of rest you are getting, and set the white noise function if you need a little help. Bonus: it also can track your fitness and food throughout the day.

Headspace—Touted as a gym for the mind, this app offers 2-minute to 1-hour-long meditation programs and exercises aimed at helping you drop into mindfulness at any point during the day.

Think Dirty—Our skin is our largest organ, and it ingests everything it comes into contact with. Many of the lotions and potions we use contain harmful chemical ingredients, but this app aims to help you shop for safer choices at the drug store and makeup counter.

ShopWell—Created by registered dietitian and nutritionist Lara Felton, this app helps you make healthier choices when at the grocery store while tracking your allergies and keeping your health goals in mind.

AFAR—This experiential guide offers a look into 50+ countries with categories such as "must-do experiences," "best of hotels," and "three-day itineraries." Offering choices from budget to luxury, it allows you to get out of your hotel room even if you haven't planned your trip in advance.

In the end, whether at home, at work, or on the road, wellness is a balance. Maintaining that balance for yourself—within yourself—enables you to extend that same balance in all directions, to everything you do. Wellness in not determined by one stand-alone factor. In fact, as you get further along your wellness journey, you'll realize just how interconnected everything is, how the actions you take affect those around you and impact the direction in which your path forks. As you begin to master your craft, help yourself to stay on the path by remembering 5 words that not only bring you back to your center, but also set you up for success: Breathe. Move. Mindful. Experience. Nourish.

This carefully researched and personally vetted book provides you the tools you need to create a solid foundation and learn ways to maximum wellness in your life. Remember, start small and choose to focus on the areas that work for you at this time. Find your routine, work it, and enjoy the benefits for years to come. If you fail, pick yourself up and try again. Your body, mind, and life will thank you for it again and again for years to come. Everyone needs a compelling reason to find their road to wellness. You already have yours. You picked up this book.

LIVING WELL ON THE ROAD CHECKLISTS

EVALUATE YOUR SLEEP

Think you have a sleep problem? Take stock of these daily routines so you can discuss them with your health-care professional.

- When you go to bed and get up during workdays:
- When you go to bed and get up during nonworkdays:
- What is your exercise routine:
- How much alcohol, caffeine, and/or tobacco you consume weekly:
- What medications (prescribed and over-the-counter) do you take:
- Do you wake up in the middle of the night? Why:
- How often do you have trouble sleeping in a week:
- Most recent significant life events:
- Describe your bedroom setup:
- Describe your presleep routine:

CREATE A SLEEP ROUTINE

Create a nightly sleep routine to ensure that no matter where in the world you find yourself, you're setting up for a good night's sleep.

- Set your alarm for the same time every morning.
- Get some kind of physical activity every day.
- Curb your food and drink intake a few hours before bed.
- Stop working 2 to 3 hours before bed.
- Cut your exposure to bright and blue light 1-hour before you plan to be asleep.
- Form a prebed routine: take a bath, wash your face, brush your teeth, journal; anything that signals to your body it's time to start slowing down.
- Keep the room at a cool temperature; between 60 and 67 degrees is recommended.
- Kick your pets (and/or kids) out of bed.

3-MINUTE CALMING EXERCISE

- Find a comfortable seated position with your feet grounded on the floor.
- Close your eyes.
- Inhale to the count of three, 1–2–3.
- Exhale to the count of three, 1–2–3.
- Repeat this a few times then increase your inhale and exhale by a count of one so now it's: Inhale 1–2–3–4, Exhale 1–2–3–4.
- You can continuously increase your inhale and exhale evenly as you wish.
- Eventually after consistent practice, you'll only need 1 minute to reap the calming benefits of this breath exercise.

2 MINUTES TO REFOCUS (BEST DONE IN FLAT SHOES OR BAREFOOT)

- Stand up straight.
- Close your eyes.
- Take a deep inhale and exhale.
- Roll your head to the right 3 times.
- Roll your head to the left 3 times.
- Roll your shoulders back 3 times.
- Roll your shoulders forward 3 times.

- On an inhale, stretch your arms up toward the ceiling, look up.
- On an exhale, interlace your hands behind your back and stretch your chest open.
- Once more, inhale and stretch up, then exhale, interlace your hands behind your back, and imagine your chest expanding.
- Place your left hand on your hip and stretch your right arm up and over your head toward the left, bending at the left waist.
- Place your right hand on your hip and stretch your left arm up and over your head toward the right, bending at the right waist.
- Repeat once more: bend toward the left, then right.
- Gently bend your knees and fold your torso down toward the floor until your hands touch, continuing to bend your knees as much as you have to.
- Inhale and exhale for 3 breaths.
- Slowly roll up to stand up straight.
- Close your eyes.
- Take a deep inhale and exhale.

ITEMS FOR YOUR GROCERY CART

Keep your house full of some healthy anti-inflammatory foods, which offer better meal and snack options. Load your cart with:

- **Raw Vegetables**: broccoli, carrots, and celery
- **Berries**: blueberries, blackberries, and strawberries
- **Leafy Greens**: spinach, kale, and swiss chard
- **Healthy Fats**: almonds, walnuts, and avocados
- **Whole Grains**: buckwheat, lentils, and steel-cut oats
- **Spices**: ginger, turmeric, and cinnamon

52-WEEK WELLNESS IMPLEMENTATION IN MANAGEABLE SEGMENTS

The definition of insanity is doing the same thing over and over and expecting different results. In order to achieve new, healthier results, it is best to start simple, get into a groove, and build from there. If you feel you've failed, start over or skip to subsequent weeks to find the pattern that allows you to be successful.

WEEK 1-3: Take the stairs and/or park far away from your destination, walking whenever possible.

WEEK 4-6: Start every day with a calming breath exercise.

WEEK 7-9: Turn all devices off 1 hour before bedtime.

WEEK 10-12: Plan a vacation.

WEEK 13-15: Find a tribe to support your change.

WEEK 16-18: Commit to having a plate full of more vegetables than anything else.

WEEK 19-21: Stop working/checking emails after 9pm.

WEEK 22-24: Put an away message on your email and take a true vacation.

WEEK 25-27: Work your sleep routine.

WEEK 28-30: Reduce your alcohol and/or sugar intake.

WEEK 31-33: Make over your workspace in a way that benefits your wellness.

WEEK 34-36: Prioritize fitness—at least 3 sessions a week (5 if you already have a routine).

WEEK 37-39: Celebrate your successes.

WEEK 40-42: Cook more meals at home than you eat out.

WEEK 43-45: Schedule in breaks at work, where you stand or walk, and stick to them.

WEEK 46-48: Pack lunch and healthy snacks for work.

WEEK 49-52: Smile at everyone you meet before you begin to talk.

WELLNESS PACKING LIST

If you're a frequent traveler, keep these items prepacked in your suitcase so you don't have to spend time collecting them.

- Photos of your passport, license, and credit cards (on your smartphone or tablet)
- Sneakers or walking shoes
- Exercise clothing

- Refillable water bottle
- Activated charcoal
- Antibacterial wipes or essential oils
- Antiviral skin salve
- Sleeping mask
- Long scarf to double as a blanket
- Travel pillow
- Natural laundry detergent
- Yoga Tune Up Balls
- Bathing suit

JET LAG KILLERS

Pretravel Routine

Start with a 24-hour routine and once perfected, expand it to 48 hours.

- Set your vacation away email to send 48 hours before your departure.
- Let clients and coworkers know you will not be checking your email while away. (Remove email access from your phone if necessary.)
- Check in for your flight at the 24-hour mark to confirm your seat assignment.
- Get a full 7-9 hours sleep the night before you depart.
- Get in a sweaty workout before you board the plane.
- Drink a low-sugar vegetable smoothie to optimize nutrition.
- Enjoy a high-quality, low-carb, healthy fat "last" meal.
- Drink a glass of water for every hour of flight time ahead.
- Pack snacks to avoid airplane food.
- Start your bedtime routine before you head to the airport.
- Drink a relaxing tea an hour before takeoff.

In-Flight Wellness

- Board early to make sure there's room for your luggage.

- Make these items easily accessible: water, eye mask, earplugs, scarf, and travel pillow.
- Clean armrests, tray tables, and the window area with anti-bacterial wipes or essential oils.
- Apply antibacterial salve to wrists, chest, and upper lip.
- Use a scarf to double as a blanket and pillow barrier.
- Treat in-flight time as self-care: read, write, watch movies, sleep, etc.
- Drink enough to use the bathroom.
- Skip the airplane food and eat your packed snacks.
- Overnight flight: Get ready for "bed" with your bedtime routine.

Arrival Routine

- Call ahead to confirm your room will be ready upon arrival.
- Unpack your bags and move in for the duration of your stay.
- Morning arrival: Work out outdoors and eat a protein-rich meal.
- Evening arrival: Head to the sauna then bed, skipping food if possible.
- Watch the first sunset and sunrise of the day to help recalibrate your circadian rhythm.
- Bonus: For a short trip, skip adjusting to a new time zone. Instead, wear sunglasses on the plane and in the mornings; sleep with an eye mask and use black-out shades to keep the light at bay at night.

WELLNESS DURING A DAY ON THE ROAD

Insert these daily wellness routines when away from home to feel better and more productive.

- Keep the blinds cracked open to wake with the sun.
- Practice breathing or meditating for 5 minutes while sitting up in bed.

- Head outdoors and walk around the block (or work out) before you sit down for breakfast.
- Eat a protein-rich, low-carb first meal.
- Alternate between sitting and standing throughout the day.
- Find a way to take a 10-minute break around lunch so you can get outdoors.
- Eat a slow-paced lunch with a focus on fresh vegetables.
- Head to the bathroom or another private space for a 3-minute breathing exercise instead of having another cup of coffee.
- Reduce your alcohol intake after work.
- Find a farm-to-table dinner option.
- Wind down in a healthy way before bed (workout, sauna, shower, bedtime routine, or no electronics).

RE-INTEGRATION POST-VACATION

You've just spent some much-needed time away, yet real life awaits your return. Hold on to that changed-by-travel feeling with these simple steps:

- Consider arriving home a day or two before you have to head back to the office so you can adjust.
- If you're traveling solo, send an email home saying you can't wait to see everyone, but walking into chaos will not be beneficial for anyone. Request kids have their toys put away or ask your partner to tidy the kitchen.
- Keep your social schedule to a minimum the week following your return to help you accommodate for jet lag or the possibility of having to catch up at work.
- Don't check your phone upon landing. This is the fastest way to kill your vacation buzz as it plunges you back into the exact things you were taking a vacation from.
- Thank yourself for investing in Global Entry, as skipping lines at customs saved you a lot of headache.
- Pay it forward with a smile. Hold on to your vacation glow by putting others at ease, as they'll feed off your relaxed energy.

MINI STEPS TO SUCCESS

- Determine which habit or behavior or lifestyle component you want to change.
- Break down that big-ticket item into small daily, weekly, and monthly goals.
- Look at the financial implications of making this change.
- Every time you reach a daily, weekly, or monthly goal, celebrate in a healthy way.
- Reevaluate—can you improve your steps to more easily obtain your goals?
- Track how your life has changed as a result of meeting your goals.
- After you've reached a few mini goals, ask yourself: "Do I still want the same success, or has the goal changed?"
- Repeat until you've found your success.

DEDICATION

To Fed—without your unwavering support, none of this would be possible. Judy, Elliott, and Matt, thank you for creating and holding the foundation from which my wellness journey blossomed.

Deep gratitude and thanks to the experts who agreed to be part of this project: Alexia Brue, Melisse Guela, Tevis Trower, Richard Louv, Dr. Robin Berzin, and Dr. Ana C. Krieger. Special thanks to Andrew McCarthy for writing the foreword and sharing his travel stories that continue to inspire me. Profound gratitude to Dr. Miles Neale, who not only agreed to be interviewed for this book but whose voice and wise words helped me begin every day and held the space for me to write.

Thank you to Jennifer Forte-Cuomo, who planted the seed. Many thanks to my tireless agent Steven Harris, who was able to see outside the box and become my champion. To my editor Suzanne Staszak-Silva and the team at Rowman & Littlefield who guided me through the process.

To all my family and friends who have been cheerleaders along the way, this book exists because of your support. And while there are too many people to name, special thanks are owed to Josh and Meredith Levine, Lindsey Jarrett, Katie Jehenson, Mary Gehlhar, Mark Kiernan, Adam Walden, Ash Brown, Jill Albino, Effie Katechis, Danielle Valentino, and Victoria Harbertson.

NOTES

CHAPTER 1

1. World Health Organization, "Wellness," www.who.int/about/definition/en/print.html

2. Huth, C., et al., "Job Strain as a Risk Factor for the Onset of Type 2 Diabetes Mellitus: Findings from the MONICA/KORA Augsburg Cohort Study," *Psychosomatic Medicine* 76, 7 (September 2014): 562-68. DOI: 10.1097/PSY.0000000000000084

3. American Psychological Association, "Stress in America: Our Health at Risk," January 11, 2012. https://www.apa.org/news/press/releases/stress/2011/final-2011.pdf

4. Weil, Andrew, "Integrative Medicine: A Vital Part of the New Health Care System," Testimony Before the Committee on Health, Education, Labor, and Pensions, United States Senate, February 26, 2009.

5. Starfield, B., L. Shi, and J. Macinko, "Contribution of Primary Care to Health Systems and Health," *The Milbank Quarterly* 83, 3 (2005): 457-502.

6. American Psychological Association, "Stress in America: Our Health at Risk," January 11, 2012.

7. Schaffer, Linden, "Well on the Road Interview," 2015/2016.

8. American Psychological Association, "Stress in America: Our Health at Risk," January 11, 2012.

9. The Commonwealth Fund, "National Trend in the Cost of Employer Health Insurance Coverage," 2003-2013. http://www.commonwealthfund.org/~/media/files/publications/issue-brief/2014/dec/1793_collins_nat_premium_trends_2003_2013.pdf

10. Kaiser Family Foundation, "2014 Employer Health Benefits Survey," Kaiser/HRET, 2004–2014, September 2014.

11. The Commonwealth Fund, "National Trend in the Cost of Employer Health Insurance Coverage," 2003–2013.

12. Gallup-Healthways, "Well-Being Index," 2008.

13. Harvard School of Public Health, "Coffee by the Numbers," 2010. http://www.hsph.harvard.edu/news/multimedia-article/facts/

14. Devries, Linda K., *Insomnia: Don't Lose Sleep Over It . . . Find the Help You Need* (Chicago: Harold Shaw Publishers, 2000).

15. Centers for Disease Control and Prevention, "Stress at Work," National Institute of Occupational Safety and Health, 2014. https://www.cdc.gov/niosh/docs/99-101/

16. Reaney, Patricia, "Global Spa, Wellness Industry Estimated at $3.4 Trillion," *Reuters*, September 30, 2014.

17. Mark, Gloria J., and Stephen Voida, "A Pace Not Dictated by Electrons: An Empirical Study of Work Without Email," Department of Informatics, University of California, Irvine. https://www.ics.uci.edu/gmark/home_page/research_files/chi%202012.pdf

18. Twain, Mark, *The American Claimant* (New York: Charles L. Webster and Company, 1892), 227.

19. Parry, Thomas, "Total Lost-Time Management: The Link between Absence and Presenteeism," *Integrated Benefits Institute*, June 2008.

20. Global Wellness Institute, "Statistics & Facts." http://www.globalwellnessinstitute.org/statistics-and-facts/

21. Berry, Leonard, Ann Mirabito, and William Baun, "What's the Hard Return on Employee Wellness Programs?" *Harvard Business Review*, December 2010. https://hbr.org/2010/12/whats-the-hard-return-on-employee-wellness-programs

22. Mattke, Soeren, et al., "Workplace Wellness Program Study," *RAND Health*, 2013.

23. Berry, Leonard, Ann Mirabito, and William Baun, "What's the Hard Return on Employee Wellness Programs?" *Harvard Business Review*, December 2010.

24. Schaffer, Linden, "Well on the Road Interview," 2015/2016.

25. Fodor, Kate, "25 Surprising Ways Stress Affects Your Health," *Health*, www.health.com/health/gallery/0,,20642595,00.html

26. Careerbuilder Survey, "Teachers, Engineers and Scientists among Most Likely to Gain Weight on the Job," May 2013. Conducted Online within the U.S. by Harris Interactive. http://www.careerbuilder.com/share/aboutus/pressreleasesdetail.aspx?sd=5/30/2013&id=pr760&ed=12/31/2013

27. Groesz, Lisa, et al., "What Is Eating You? Stress and the Drive to Eat," *Appetite* 58, 2 (April 2012): 717-21.

28. McMullen, Tom, "Enabling, Engaging, & Rewarding Employees," *Hay Group*, Mexico City, April 6, 2011.

29. Stewart, Walter F., et al., "Cost of Lost Productive Work Time among U.S. Workers with Depression," *JAMA* 289, 23 (June 18, 2003): 3135-44.

30. Walker, Rob, "Jeff Bezos, Amazon.Com, Because 'Optimism Is Essential,'" *Inc. Magazine*, 2004. http://www.inc.com/magazine/20040401/25bezos.html

31. "Millennial Consumer Study 2015," *Elite Daily*, January 19, 2015. http://Elitedaily.Com/News/Business/Elite-Daily-Millennial-Consumer-Survey-2015/

32. Goldman Sachs, "Millennial Impact Study," 2014. http://www.goldmansachs.com/our-thinking/pages/millennials/

33. American Psychological Association, "Stress in America: Our Health at Risk," January 11, 2012.

34. Lerman, Katrina, "Healthcare Without Borders: How Millennials Are Reshaping Health and Wellness," *Communispace*, 2014. https://healthcaresocialmedia.files. wordpress.com/2014/11/how-millennials-are-reshaping-digital-health.png

35. Lerman, Katrina, "Healthcare Without Borders: How Millennials are Reshaping Health and Wellness," *Communispace*, 2014.

36. Lerman, Katrina, "Healthcare Without Borders: How Millennials are Reshaping Health and Wellness," *Communispace*, 2014.

37. His Holiness the Dalai Lama, *The Path to Tranquility: Daily Meditations* (New York: Penguin Books, 1998).

38. American Psychological Association, "Stress in America: Our Health at Risk," January 11, 2012.

39. Young, Richard and Jennifer DeVoe, "Who Will Have Health Insurance in the Future? An Updated Projection," *Annals of Family Medicine* 10 (2012): 156-62. DOI: 10.1370/afm.1348

CHAPTER 2

1. Xie, L., et al., "Sleep Initiated Fluid Flux Drives Metabolite Clearance from the Adult Brain," *Science*, October 18, 2013. DOI: 10.1126/Science.1241224

2. Graves, Ginny, "10 Strategies for a More Restful Night's Sleep," *Allure Magazine* 9, 11 (2008): 1195-200.

3. Drake, C. J., "Caffeine Effects on Sleep Taken 0, 3, or 6 Hours Before Going to Bed," *Journal of Clinical Sleep Medicine* 9, 11 (November 15, 2013).

4. Graves, Ginny, "10 Strategies for a More Restful Night's Sleep," *Allure Magazine*, 2008.

5. Richter, Jean Paul, trans., "The Notebooks of Leonardo Da Vinci," 1888, www.gutenberg.org/cache/epub/5000/pg5000.html

6. Carlson, Emily, "Resetting Our Clocks: New Details about How the Body Tells Time," *NIH—National Institute of General Medical Sciences*, March 2014.

7. Gottlieb, D. J., et al., "Novel Loci Associated with Usual Sleep Duration: The CHARGE Consortium Genome-Wide Association Study," *Molecular Psychiatry* 20, 10 (October 2015): 1232–39. DOI: 10.1038/Mp.2014.133. Epub December 2, 2014

8. Hamilton, Elizabeth, "Feel Groggy in the Mornings? Here's How to Wake Up Refreshed," *Dallas Morning News*, February 16, 2015.

9. Roenneberg, Till, "Is Light-at-Night a Health Risk Factor or a Health Risk Predictor?" *Chronobiology International: The Journal of Biological and Medical Rhythm Research* 26, 6 (2009). DOI: 10.3109/07420520903223984

10. Vaze, K. M., and V. K. Sharma, "On the Adaptive Significance of Circadian Clocks for Their Owners," *Chronobiology International* 30, 4 (May 2013): 413–33. DOI: 10.3109/07420528.2012.754457. Epub March 4, 2013

11. Turek, F. W., and P. C. Zee, eds., "The Impact of Changes in Night-length (Scotoperiod) on Human Sleep," in *Neurobiology of Sleep and Circadian Rhythms* (New York: Marcel Dekker, 1999), 263–85.

12. Akerstedt, T., et al., "Awakening from Sleep," *Sleep Medicine Reviews* 6, 4 (2002), www.ncbi.nlm.nih.gov/pubmed/12531132

13. Eng, Monica, "Light from Electronic Screens at Night Linked to Sleep Loss," *Chicago Tribune*, July 8, 2012.

14. Chang, Anne-Marie, "Evening Use of Light-Emitting Ereaders Negatively Affects Sleep, Circadian Timing, and Next-Morning Alertness," National Institutes of Health, Brigham and Women's Hospital, January 27, 2015.

15. Stevens, Richard, "The Key to Feeling Well Rested Isn't Just the Amount of Time You Sleep," *Business Insider*, April 6, 2015.

16. Wright, H. R., "Effect of Light Wavelength on Suppression and Phase Delay of the Melatonin Rhythm," *Chronobiology International* 18, 5 (September 2001): 801–8.

17. Chang, Anne-Marie, "Evening Use of Light-Emitting Ereaders Negatively Affects Sleep, Circadian Timing, and Next-Morning Alertness," January 27, 2015.

18. Chang, Anne-Marie, "Evening Use of Light-Emitting Ereaders Negatively Affects Sleep, Circadian Timing, and Next-Morning Alertness," January 27, 2015.

19. New York Blue Light Symposium, "Welcome Message," June 2015. http://blue-light.biz/2isbls/img/Panf-2isbls.pdf

20. Blask, David, et al., "Light Pollution: Adverse Health Effects of Nighttime Lighting," Action of the AMA House of Delegates 2012, Annual Meeting: Council on Science and Public Health Report 4. http://www.atmob.org/library/resources/AMA%20Health%20Effects%20Light%20at%20Night.pdf

21. IARC, "Painting, Firefighting, and Shiftwork: IARC Monographs on the Evaluation of Carcinogenic Risks to Humans," Vol. 98. Lyon, France: International Agency for Research on Cancer, Working Group on the Evaluation of Carcinogenic Risks to Humans, 2007.

22. Jones, Jeffrey M., "In U.S., 40% Get Less than Recommended Amount of Sleep," *Gallup*, December 19, 2013. http://www.gallup.com/poll/166553/less-recommended-amount-sleep.aspx

23. Harvard Medical School, "Insomnia: Restoring Restful Sleep. The Family Health Guide," *Harvard Medical Publications*, March 2009.

24. Barnes, Christopher M., "Sleep-deprived People Are More Likely to Cheat," *Harvard Business Review*, May 31, 2013.

25. Konnikova, Maria, "Why Can't We Fall Asleep?" *New Yorker*, July 7, 2015.

26. Czeisler, Charles, "A Sleep Epidemic," *TED Talk*, 2001. https://www.youtube.com/watch?v=p4UxLpoNCxU

27. Borzykowski, Bryan, "Successful Executives and the Four-hour Sleep Myth," *Harvard Business Review*, October 12, 2012. https://hbr.org/2012/10/if-youre-too-busy-to-meditate.html

28. Belenky, G., "Patterns of Performance Degradation and Restoration During Sleep Restriction and Subsequent Recovery: A Sleep Dose Response Study," *Journal of Sleep Research* 12 (March 2003): 1–12.

29. Fryer, Bronwyn, "Sleep Deficit: The Performance Killer," *Harvard Business Review*, October 2006.

30. National Heart, Lung, and Blood Institute, "Why Is Sleep Important?" February 2012. http://www.nhlbi.nih.gov/health/health-topics/topics/sdd/why

31. Society for Neuroscience, "Sleep-deprived Brains Alternate Between Normal Activity and 'Power Failure,'" May 2008.

32. Fryer, Bronwyn, "Sleep Deficit: The Performance Killer," *Harvard Business Review*, October 2006.

33. Zevon, Warren, "I'll Sleep When I'm Dead." *Warren Zevon*. Asylum Records, 1976.

34. Rechtschaffen, Allan and Bernard Bergmann, "Sleep Deprivation in the Rat: An Update of the 1989 Paper," *Sleep* 25, 1 (2002): 18–24.

35. Johnson, Carla, "Preventing Colds May Be as Easy as Vitamin Zzz Updated," Associated Press, January 2009.

36. Kahan, V., "Can Poor Sleep Affect Skin Integrity?" *Medical Hypotheses* 75, 6 (December 2010): 535–37. DOI: 10.1016/J.Mehy.2010.07.018. Epub August 1, 2010. http://www.ncbi.nlm.nih.gov/pubmed/20678867

37. Czeisler, Charles, "A Sleep Epidemic," *TED Talk*, 2001.

38. Lewine, Howard, "Too Little Sleep, and Too Much, Affect Memory," *Harvard Health Blog*, May 2014. http://www.health.harvard.edu/blog/little-sleep-much-affect-memory-201405027136

39. Harvard Medical School, "Sleep and Disease Risk," December 2007. http://healthysleep.med.harvard.edu/healthy/matters/consequences/sleep-and-disease-risk

40. Knutson, K. L., A. M. Ryden, V. A. Mander, and E. Van Cauter, "Role of Sleep Duration and Quality in the Risk and Severity of Type 2 Diabetes Mellitus," *Archives of Internal Medicine* 166 (2006): 1768–64.

41. Harris, Shelby Freedman, "6 Ways Sleep Makes Your Life Better," *The Huffington Post Healthy Living*, September 14, 2014. http://www.huffingtonpost.com/2014/09/14/benefits-of-sleep_n_5799214.html

42. Nielsen, Tore, "Dreams of the Rarebit Fiend: Food and Diet as Instigators of Bizarre and Disturbing Dreams," *Frontiers in Psychology*, February 17, 2015. http://dx.doi.org/10.3389/fpsyg.2015.00047

43. Ryu, Ja Young, "Association Between Body Size Phenotype and Sleep Duration: Korean National Health and Nutrition Examination Survey V," December 1, 2014.

44. Colwell, Christopher, "Eating During Sleep Periods May Impair Memory," presented at Neuroscience 2014, the Annual Meeting of the Society for Neuroscience.

45. Tierney, John, "Do You Suffer from Decision Fatigue?" *New York Times Magazine*, August 17, 2011.

46. Tierney, John, "Do You Suffer from Decision Fatigue?" *New York Times Magazine*, August 17, 2011.

47. Anwar, Yasmin, "Sleep Loss Linked to Psychiatric Disorders," *UC Berkeley*, October 22, 2015. http://www.berkeley.edu/news/media/releases/2007/10/22_sleeploss.shtml

48. Anwar, Yasmin, "Sleep Loss Linked to Psychiatric Disorders," *UC Berkeley*, October 22, 2015.

49. National Sleep Foundation, "Sleep-Wake Cycle: Its Physiology and Impact on Health," 2006. https://sleepfoundation.org/sites/default/files/SleepWakeCycle.pdf

50. Altena, Ellemarije, et al., "Reduced Orbitofrontal and Parietal Gray Matter in Chronic Insomnia: A Voxel-Based Morphometric Study," *Biolog-*

ical Psychiatry Journal 67, 2 (September 2009). http://dx.doi.org/10.1016/j.biopsych.2009.08.003

51. Steinbeck, John, *Sweet Thursday* (New York: Viking Press, 1954).

52. Schaffer, Linden, "Well on the Road Interview," 2015/2016.

53. Cutrone, Carolyn and Max Nisen, "19 Successful People Who Barely Sleep," *Business Insider*, September 2012.

54. Borzykowski, Bryan. "Successful Executives and the Four-Hour Sleep Myth," *Harvard Business Review*, October 12, 2012.

55. Centers for Disease Control and Prevention, "Short Sleep Duration among Workers—United States, 2010," *Morbidity and Mortality Weekly Report* 61, 16 (April 27, 2012): 281-85.

56. Kessler, R. C., et al., "Insomnia and the Performance of U.S. Workers: Results from the America Insomnia Survey," *Sleep* 34, 9 (September 1, 2011): 1161-71. DOI: 10.5665/SLEEP.1230

57. Barnes, Christopher M., "Sleep-deprived People Are More Likely to Cheat," *Harvard Business Review*, May 31, 2013.

58. Lockley, Steven W., et al., "Effect of Reducing Interns' Weekly Work Hours on Sleep and Attentional Failures," *The New England Journal of Medicine* 351 (October 28, 2004): 1829-37. DOI: 10.1056/NEJMoa041404

59. McGregor, Jenna, "The Average Worker Loses 11 Days of Productivity Each Year Due to Insomnia, and Companies Are Taking Notice," *Washington Post*, July 30, 2015.

60. Basner, Mathias, et al., "Sociodemographic Characteristics and Waking Activities and Their Role in the Timing and Duration of Sleep," *Sleep* 37, 12 (2014). http://dx.doi.org/10.5665/sleep.4238

61. Evans, Lisa, "Want More Sleep (and Better Productivity)? Work from Home," *Entrepreneur Magazine*, February 17, 2015.

62. Korn, Melissa, "Smartphones Make You Tired and Unproductive, Study Says," *Wall Street Journal*, February 6, 2014.

63. Huffington, Arianna, "My Q and A with Michael Breus, aka the Sleep Doctor," *The Huffington Post*, September 8, 2015. http://www.huffingtonpost.com/arianna-huffington/my-q-and-a-with-michael-breus-aka-the-sleep-doctor_b_8104520.html

64. Blanaru, Monica, "The Effects of Music Relaxation and Muscle Relaxation Techniques on Sleep Quality and Emotional Measures among Individuals with Posttraumatic Stress Disorder," *Mental Illness Journal* 4, 2 (July 26, 2012): E13.

65. Afonso, R. F., "Yoga Decreases Insomnia in Postmenopausal Women: A Randomized Clinical Trial," *Menopause* 19, 2 (February 2012): 186-93. DOI: 10.1097/Gme.0b013e318228225f

66. Puhan, Milo A., "Didgeridoo Playing as Alternative Treatment for Obstructive Sleep Apnea Syndrome: Randomized Controlled Trial," *British Medical Journal*, February 2006.

67. Lovato, Nicole, "Evaluation of a Brief Treatment Program of Cognitive Behavior Therapy for Insomnia in Older Adults," *Sleep* 37, 1. http://dx.doi.org/10.5665/sleep.3320

68. Parker, Ian, "The Big Sleep," *New Yorker*, December 9, 2013. http://www.newyorker.com/magazine/2013/12/09/the-big-sleep-2

69. Fryer, Bronwyn, "Sleep Deficit: The Performance Killer," *Harvard Business Review*, October 2006.

70. Parker, Ian, "The Big Sleep," *New Yorker*, December 9, 2013.

CHAPTER 3

1. Milne, A. A., *When We Were Very Young* (New York: Puffin Books, 1924), 86.

2. Myers, Jonathan, "Exercise and Cardiovascular Health," *American Heart Association*, 2003. DOI: 10.1161/01.CIR.0000048890.59383.8D

3. Fisher, R., et al., "Stand Up For Health—Avoiding Sedentary Behaviour Might Lengthen Your Telomeres: Secondary Outcomes from a Physical Activity RCT in Older People," *British Journal of Sports Medicine* 48, 19 (2014): 1407-9.

4. Merchant, Nilofer, "Got a Meeting? Take a Walk," *TED*, 2013, www.ted.com/talks/nilofer_merchant_got_a_meeting_take_a_walk?language=en

5. Yue, Pengying, "Neck/Shoulder Pain and Low Back Pain among School Teachers in China, Prevalence and Risk Factors," *BMC Public Health* 12 (2012): 789. DOI:10.1186/1471-2458-12-789

6. Lin, F., "Effect of Different Sitting Postures on Lung Capacity, Expiratory Flow, and Lumbar Lordosis," *Archives of Physical Medicine and Rehabilitation* 87, 4 (April 2006): 504-9.

7. Jensen, Eric, *Learning with the Body in Mind* (Thousand Oaks, CA: Corwin Press, 2000).

8. Spain, Erin, "Even Physically Active Women Sit Too Much," October 2012, www.northwestern.edu/newscenter/stories/2012/10/even-physically-active-women-sit-too-much.html

9. University of London, "New Study Reveals How Changes in Lifestyle Are Contributing to Dramatic Rise in Obesity," August 28, 2015.

10. Ekelund, Ulf, et al., "Physical Activity and All-Cause Mortality Across Levels of Overall and Abdominal Adiposity in European Men and Women: The European Prospective Investigation into Cancer and Nutrition Study (EPIC)," *American Journal of Clinical Exercise* 2015. DOI: 10.3945/Ajcn.114.100065

11. Kohl, Harold W., "The Pandemic of Physical Inactivity: Global Action for Public Health," *The Lancet*, July 18, 2012. http://dx.doi.org/10.1016/s0140-6736(12)60898-8

12. Centers for Disease Control and Prevention, "Physical Activity—Glossary of Terms," June 2015.

13. Lewis, Steven and Charles H. Hennekens, "Regular Physical Activity: Forgotten Benefits," *The American Journal of Medicine* 129, 2 (2016). DOI: 10.1016/J.Amjmed.2015.07.016

14. Kohl, Harold W., "The Pandemic of Physical Inactivity: Global Action for Public Health," *The Lancet* 380, 9838 (2012).

15. Lewis, Steven, and Charles H. Hennekens, "Regular Physical Activity," *The American Journal of Medicine* 129, 2 (2015).

16. Yang, Quanhe, "Morbidity and Mortality Weekly Report (MMWR), Center for Disease Control, Vital Signs: Predicted Heart Age and Racial Disparities in Heart Age among U.S. Adults at the State Level," September 1, 2015.

17. Booth, Frank W., "Lack of Exercise Is a Major Cause of Chronic Diseases," *Comprehensive Physiology* 2, 2 (April 2012): 1143–211. DOI: 10.1002/Cphy.C110025 Pmcid: Pmc4241367 Nihmsid: Nihms603913

18. Centers for Disease Control and Prevention, "Heart Disease Fact Sheet," November 30, 2015.

19. Myers, Jonathan, "Exercise and Cardiovascular Health," *American Heart Association*, 2003.

20. Myers, Jonathan, "Exercise and Cardiovascular Health," *American Heart Association*, 2003.

21. Mercola, Joseph, "This Is What Happens to Your Body When You Exercise," *Peak Fitness*, September 20, 2013.

22. Booth, Frank W., "Lack of Exercise Is a Major Cause of Chronic Diseases," *Comprehensive Physiology* 2, 2 (April 2012): 1143–211.

23. Parajuli, Ashutosh, "Bone's Responses to Mechanical Loading Are Impaired in Type 1 Diabetes," *Bone*. Published online: July 13, 2015. DOI: http://dx.doi.org/10.1016/j.bone.2015.07.012

24. Parajuli, Ashutosh, "Bone's Responses to Mechanical Loading Are Impaired in Type 1 Diabetes," *Bone*. Published online: July 13, 2015.

25. Booth, Frank W., "Lack of Exercise Is a Major Cause of Chronic Diseases," *Comprehensive Physiology* 2, 2 (April 2012): 1143–211.

26. Gram, Martin, et al., "Two Weeks of One-leg Immobilization Decreases Skeletal Muscle Respiratory Capacity Equally in Young and Elderly Men," *Experimental Gerontology* 58, 10 (2014): 269–78.

27. Mayo Clinic, "HDL Cholesterol: How to Boost Your 'Good' Cholesterol," November 2012. http://www.mayoclinic.org/diseases-conditions/high-blood-cholesterol/in-depth/hdl-cholesterol/art-20046388?pg=2

28. Reynolds, Gretchen, "Weighing the Evidence on Exercise," *New York Times Magazine*, April 16, 2010.

29. Maclean, P. S., "Regular Exercise Attenuates the Metabolic Drive to Regain Weight after Longterm Weight Loss," *American Journal of Physiology—Regulatory, Integrative and Comparative Physiology* 297, 3 (September 2009): R793802. DOI: 10.1152/Ajpregu.00192.2009. Epub July 8, 2009

30. Higgins, Janine A., "Resistant Starch and Exercise Independently Attenuate Weight Regain on a High Fat Diet in a Rat Model of Obesity," *Nutrition & Metabolism* 8 (July 7, 2011): 49. DOI: 10.1186/1743-7075-8 -4907

31. Lee, I-Min, "Physical Activity and Weight Gain Prevention," *JAMA* 303, 12 (2010): 1173-79. DOI:10.1001/Jama.2010.312

32. Weir, Kirsten, "The Exercise Effect," *American Psychological Association* 42, 11 (December 2011). http://www.apa.org/monitor/2011/12/exercise.aspx

33. Weir, Kirsten, "The Exercise Effect," *American Psychological Association* 42, 11 (December 2011).

34. Hoffman, Benson M., et al., "Exercise and Pharmacotherapy in Patients with Major Depression: One-year Follow-up of the Smile Study," *Psychosomatic Medicine* 73, 2 (February–March 2011): 127-33. DOI: 10.1097/Psy.0b013e31820433a5. Epub December 10, 2010

35. Anxiety and Depression Association of America, "Exercise for Stress and Anxiety," July 2014, www.adaa.org/living-with-anxiety/managing-anxiety/exercise-stress-and-anxiety

36. Chrysohoou, C., "High Intensity, Interval Exercise Improves Quality of Life of Patients with Chronic Heart Failure: A Randomized Controlled Trial," *Quarterly Journal of Medicine* 107 (2014): 25-32. DOI: 10.1093/qjmed/hct194. Advance Access Publication, September 30, 2013.

37. Bromanfulks, J. J., "Effects of Aerobic Exercise on Anxiety Sensitivity," *Behaviour Research and Therapy* 42, 2 (2004): 125-36.

38. Booth, Frank W., "Lack of Exercise Is a Major Cause of Chronic Diseases," *Comprehensive Physiology* 2, 2 (April 2012): 1143-211.

39. Booth, Frank W., "Lack of Exercise Is a Major Cause of Chronic Diseases," *Comprehensive Physiology* 2, 2 (April 2012): 1143-211.

40. Balasubramaniam, M., S. Telles, and P. M. Doraiswamy, "Yoga on Our Minds: A Systematic Review of Yoga for Neuropsychiatric Disorders," *Frontiers in Psychiatry* 3 (2013): 117. DOI: 10.3389/Fpsyt.2012.00117

41. National Center for Complementary and Integrative Health, "Use of Complementary Health Approaches in the U.S.," February 2015. https://nccih.nih.gov/research/statistics/nhis/2012/mind-body/yoga

42. Mercola, Dr., Joseph, "This Is What Happens to Your Body When You Exercise," *Peak Fitness*, September 20, 2013.

43. Wang, Q., et al., "Voluntary Exercise Counteracts Aβ25-35-induced Memory Impairment in Mice," *Behavioural Brain Research* 256 (2013): 618–25. DOI:10.1016/J.Bbr.2013.09.024

44. Erickson, Kirk I., "Exercise Training Increases Size of Hippocampus and Improves Memory," *Proceedings of the National Academy of Sciences* 108, 7 (2011): 3017–22. DOI: 10.1073/Pnas.1015950108

45. Hopkins, M. E., "Differential Effects of Acute and Regular Physical Exercise on Cognition and Affect," *Neuroscience* 215 (July 26, 2012): 59–68. DOI: 10.1016/j.neuroscience.2012.04.056. Epub April 30, 2012

46. Gow, Alan J., "Neuroprotective Lifestyles and the Aging Brain," *Neurology* 79, 17 (October 23, 2012): 1802–8. DOI: http://dx.doi.org/10.1212/WNL.0b013e3182703fd2

47. Bidwell, Allie, "Study: Physical Fitness Linked to Brain Fitness," *U.S. News & World Report*, August 19, 2014.

48. Passos, G. S., "Effects of Moderate Aerobic Exercise Training on Chronic Primary Insomnia," *Sleep Medicine* 12, 10 (December 2011): 1018127. DOI: 10.1016/J.Sleep.2011.02.007

49. Mayo Clinic Staff, "Exercise: 7 Benefits of Regular Physical Activity," February 2014. http://www.mayoclinic.org/healthy-lifestyle/fitness/in-depth/exercise/art-20048389

50. Mayo Clinic Staff, "Exercise: 7 Benefits of Regular Physical Activity," February 2014.

51. Ekelund, Ulf, et. al., "Physical Activity and All-Cause Mortality Across Levels of Overall and Abdominal Adiposity in European Men and Women: The European Prospective Investigation into Cancer and Nutrition Study (EPIC)," *American Journal of Clinical Exercise*, 2015.

52. Sifferlin, Alexandra, "Mind Your Reps: Exercise, Especially Weight Lifting, Helps Keep the Brain Sharp," *Time Magazine*, July 16, 2012.

53. Fahkry, Tony, *The Power to Navigate Your Life* (Victoria, Australia: Heart Space Publications, 2014).

54. Faux, Zeke, "Sweaty Wall Streeters Skip Booze for Spinclass Meetings," *Bloomberg Business*, July 18, 2013.

55. Coulson, J. C., J. McKenna, and M. Field, "Exercising at Work and Self-Reported Work Performance," *International Journal of Workplace Health Management* 1, 3 (2008): 176–97.

56. Coulson, J. C., J. McKenna, and M. Field, "Exercising at Work and Self-reported Work Performance," *International Journal of Workplace Health Management* 1, 3 (2008): 176–97.

57. Coulson, J. C., J. McKenna, and M. Field, "Exercising at Work and Self-reported Work Performance," *International Journal of Workplace Health Management* 1, 3 (2008): 176–97.

58. Schaffer, Linden, "Well on the Road Interview," 2015/2016.

59. Meltzer, Marisa, "Why Fitness Classes Are Making You Go Broke," *Racked*, June 10, 2015. http://www.racked.com/2015/6/10/8748149/fitness-class-costs

60. Robbins, Liz, "Great Workout, Forget the View," *New York Times*, February 18, 2009.

61. Neiger, Chris, "9 Facts You Didn't Know about Wearable Technology," *The Motley Fool*, February 15, 2016. http://www.fool.com/investing/general/2016/02/15/9-facts-you-didnt-know-about-wearable-technology.aspx

62. Mintel, "Fitness Fuels US Consumer Desire for Wearable Tech With Sales Increasing 186% in 2015," January 2016, www.idc.com/getdoc.jsp?containerid=prus40846515

63. "IDC Forecasts Worldwide Shipments of Wearables to Surpass 200 Million in 2019, Driven by Strong Smartwatch Growth," *IDC Worldwide Quarterly*, December 17, 2015.

64. Murphy, Margi, "Why Intel's Latest Purchase and Fitbit's £3.8bn Valuation Prove Wearables Aren't a Fad," *Techworld*, June 2015. http://www.techworld.com/wearables/wearables-are-not-fad-why-intels-latest-purchase-fitbits-ipo-are-proof-3616271/

65. Acquity Group, "2014 State of the Internet of Things Study," Acquity Group. http://www.acquitygroup.com/News-Andideas/Thought-Leadership/Article/Detail/Acquity-Group-2014-Internet-Of-Things-Study

66. Yang Bai, et al., "Comparison of Different Activity Monitors," *Medicine and Science in Sports & Exercise*, August 2015.

67. Goldman Sachs, "Millennials: Coming of Age," www.goldmansachs.com/our-thinking/pages/millennials/

68. Schaffer, Linden, "Well on the Road Interview," 2015/2016.

CHAPTER 4

1. Lipman, Frank, "How Do I Stay Calm with All the Stress in My Life?" Blog, January 4, 2011, www.drfranklipman.com

2. World Bank Statistic, http://data.worldbank.org/indicator/SP.DYN.LE00.IN

3. National Institutes of Mental Health, "Any Anxiety Disorder Among Adults," www.nimh.nih.gov/health/statistics/prevalence/file_148008.pdf

4. Centers for Disease Control and Prevention, "Chronic Diseases: The Power to Prevent, the Call to Control: At a Glance 2009," 2009.

5. Fryer, Bronwyn, "Are You Working Too Hard?" *Harvard Business Review*, November 2005.

6. O'Brien, Jennifer, "UCSF Study on Multitasking Reveals Switching Glitch in Aging Brain," 2011. https://www.ucsf.edu/news/2011/04/9676/ucsf-study-multitasking-reveals-switching-glitch-aging-brain

7. Hallowell, Edward, "Overloaded Circuits: Why Smart People Underperform," *Harvard Business Review*, January 2005.

8. Hallowell, Edward, "Overloaded Circuits: Why Smart People Underperform," *Harvard Business Review*, January 2005.

9. American Institute of Stress, "Workplace Stress." http://www.cdc.gov/niosh/87-111.html

10. 60 Minutes with Anderson Cooper, "Mindfulness," December 14, 2014. http://www.cbsnews.com/news/mindfulness-anderson-cooper-60-minutes/

11. Kabat-Zinn, J., L. Lipworth, R. Burney, "The Clinical Use of Mindfulness Meditation for the Self-Regulation of Chronic Pain," *Journal of Behavioral Medicine* 8, 2 (June 1985): 163–90.

12. Starr, Ringo, "Ringo Starr Receives the DLF Lifetime of Peace and Love Award," 2014. http://tmhome.com/experiences/ringo-starr-receives-a-lifetime-award/

13. Schaffer, Linden, "Well on the Road Interview," 2015/2016.

14. Desbordes, Gaëlle, "Effects of Mindful-Attention and Compassion Meditation Training on Amygdala Response to Emotional Stimuli in an Ordinary, Non-Meditative State," *Frontiers in Human Neuroscience* 6 (2012): 292. DOI: 10.3389/fnhum.2012.00292

15. Davidson, Richard J., "Buddha's Brain: Neuroplasticity and Meditation," *IEEE Signal Processing Magazine* 25, 1 (January 1, 2008): 176–74, www.ncbi.nlm.nih.gov/pmc/articles/pmc2944261

16. Motluk, Alison, "Meditation Builds Up the Brain," *New Scientist*, November 2005.

17. Luders, Eileen, Nicolas Cherbuin, and Florian Kurth, "Forever Young(er): Potential Age-Defying Effects of Long-term Meditation on Gray Matter Atrophy," *Frontiers in Psychology* 5 (2014): 1551. Published online January 21, 2015. http://journal.frontiersin.org/article/10.3389/fpsyg.2014.01551/full. DOI: 10.3389/fpsyg.2014.01551

18. McGreevey, Sue, "Eight Weeks to a Better Brain," *Harvard Gazette*, January 21, 2011.

19. Luders, Eileen, Nicolas Cherbuin, and Florian Kurth, "Forever Young(er): Potential Age-Defying Effects of Long-term Meditation on Gray Matter Atrophy," *Frontiers in Psychology* 5 (2014): 1551.

20. Wheeler, Mark, "Evidence Builds that Meditation Strengthens the Brain, UCLA Researchers Say," *UCLA Newsroom*, March 14, 2012.

21. Wheeler, Mark, "How to Build a Bigger Brain," *UCLA Newsroom*, May 12, 2009.

22. American Psychological Association, "Stress in America: Our Health at Risk," January 11, 2012. https://www.apa.org/news/press/releases/stress/2011/final-2011.pdf

23. Brendel, David, "There Are Risks to Mindfulness at Work," *Harvard Business Review*, February 11, 2015. https://hbr.org/2015/02/there-are-risks-to-mindfulness-at-work

24. Brewer, Judson, "Meditation Experience is Associated with Differences in Default Mode Network Activity and Connectivity," *Proceedings of the National Academy of Sciences of the United States of America* 108, 50 (December 13, 2011): 20254-59. DOI: 10.1073/Pnas.1112029108. Epub November 23, 2011

25. Carlson, Linda E., et al., "Mindfulness-Based Cancer Recovery and Supportive-Expressive Therapy Maintain Telomere Length Relative to Controls in Distressed Breast Cancer Survivors," *Cancer* 12, 2 (November 2014): 21-25. DOI: 10.1002/Cncr.29063

26. Jacobs, T. L., et al., "Intensive Meditation Training, Immune Cell Telomerase Activity, and Psychological Mediators," *Psychoneuroendocrinology* 36, 5 (2010): 664-81. DOI:10.1016/J.Psyneuen.2010.09.010

27. Colzato, Lorenza, "Meditate to Create: The Impact of Focused-Attention and Open-Monitoring Training on Convergent and Divergent Thinking," *Institute for Psychological Research*, Leiden University (2012).

28. Hallowell, Edward, "Overloaded Circuits: Why Smart People Underperform," *Harvard Business Review*, January 2005.

29. Schneider, Robert, "Stress Reduction in the Secondary Prevention of Cardiovascular Disease," *American Heart Association Journals*, July 16, 2012, circoutcomes.ahajournals.org/content/5/6/750.abstract

30. Brewer, J. A., "Mindfulness Training for Smoking Cessation: Results from a Randomized Controlled Trial," *Drug and Alcohol Dependence* 119, 1-2 (December 1, 2011): 72-80. DOI: 10.1016/J.Drugalcdep.2011.05.027. Epub July 1, 2011

31. Goyal, Madhav, "Mediation Programs of Psychological Stress and Well-Being," *JAMA Internal Medicine* 174, 3 (2014): 357-68.

32. Hoge, Elizabeth, "Mindfulness and Self-Compassion in Generalize Anxiety Disorder," *Evidence-based Complementary and Alternative Medicine* (2013): 34-40. DOI: 10.1155/2013/576258

33. Hoge, Elizabeth, "Mindfulness and Self-Compassion in Generalize Anxiety Disorder," *Evidence-Based Complementary and Alternative Medicine*, 2013.

34. Blanding, Michael, "National Health Costs Could Decrease if Managers Reduce Work Stress," *Harvard Business School*, January 26, 2015. http://hbswk.hbs.edu/item/7491.html

35. American Psychological Association, "Stress in America: Are Teens Adopting Adults' Stress Habits?" 2014. https://www.apa.org/news/press/releases/stress/2013/stress-report.pdf

36. American Institute of Stress, "Workplace Stress."

37. Pinsker, Joe, "Corporations' Newest Productivity Hack: Meditation," *The Atlantic*, March 10, 2015. http://www.theatlantic.com/business/archive/2015/03/corporations-newest-productivity-hack-meditation/387286/

38. Gelles, David, "The Mind Business," *Financial Times*, August 24, 2015.

39. Agnew, Harriett, "'Mindfulness' Gives Stressed-Out Bankers Something to Think About," *London Financial Times*, May 4, 2014.

40. Agnew, Harriett, "'Mindfulness' Gives Stressed-out Bankers Something to Think About," *London Financial Times*, May 4, 2014.

41. Gelles, David, "The Mind Business," *Financial Times*, August 24, 2015.

42. Burton, Katherine, "To Make a Killing on Wall Street, Start Meditating," *Bloomberg Business*, May 27, 2014.

43. Huffington, Arianna, "Mindfulness, Meditation, Wellness and Their Connection to Corporate America's Bottom Line," *The Huffington Post*, March 18, 2013.

44. Hochman, David, "Mindfulness: Getting Its Share of Attention," *The New York Times*, November 1, 2013.

45. *CBS This Morning*, "Aetna CEO Mark Bertolini on Changing Workplace and Health Care," March 26, 2015. http://www.cbsnews.com/videos/aetna-ceo-mark-bertolini-on-changing-workplace-and-health-care/

46. *CBS This Morning*, "Aetna CEO Mark Bertolini on Changing Workplace and Health Care," March 26, 2015.

47. Hochman, David, "Mindfulness: Getting Its Share of Attention," *The New York Times*, November 1, 2013.

48. Gelles, David, "The Mind Business," *Financial Times*, August 24, 2012.

49. Chopra, Deepak, "Why Wall Streeters Need to Meditate," *CNBC*, March 2015.

50. Mackenzie, Corey S., Patricia A. Poulin, and Rhonda Seidman-Carlson, "A Brief Mindfulness-Based Stress Reduction Intervention for Nurses and Nurse Aides," *Applied Nursing Research* 19 (2006): 105-9.

51. Confino, J. O., "Thich Nhat Hanh: Is Mindfulness Being Corrupted by Business and Finance?" *The Guardian*, March 28, 2014.

52. World Health Organization, "Global Status Report on Non-Communicable Diseases Chapter 5: Improving Health Care: Individual

Interventions," 1998. http://www.who.int/nmh/publications/ncd_report_chapter5.pdf

53. Becker, Gay, "Self-Care Among Chronically Ill African Americans: Culture, Health Disparities, and Health Insurance Status," *American Journal For Public Health* 94, 12 (2003): 2066-73.

54. Unterrainer, H. F., et al., "Soul Darkness? Dimensions of Religious/Spiritual Well-Being Among Mood-Disordered Inpatients Compared to Healthy Controls," *Psychopathology* 45, 5 (2012): 310-16. DOI: 10.1159/000336050

55. Koenig, H. G., "Religious Attitudes and Practices of Hospitalized Medically Ill Older Adults," *International Journal of Geriatrics Psychiatry* 13, 4 (April 1998): 213-24.

CHAPTER 5

1. Godbey, Geoffrey, "Outdoor Recreation, Health, and Wellness: Understanding and Enhancing the Relationship," *Resources for the Future*, May 2009.

2. Nesse, Randolph and George Williams, *Why We Get Sick: The New Science of Darwinian Medicine* (New York: Vintage, 1996).

3. World Health Organization, "Q&A on Artemisinin Resistance," February 2015. http://who.int/malaria/media/artemisinin_resistance _qa/en/

4. Rubinstein, A., Y. Lurie, I. Groskop, and M. Weintrob, "Cholesterol-Lowering Effects of a 10 Mg Daily Dose of Lovastatin in Patients with Initial Total Cholesterol Levels 200 to 240 Mg/Dl (5.18 to 6.21 Mmol/Liter)," *American Journal of Cardiology* 68, 11 (November 1, 1991): 1123-26. http://www.ncbi.nlm.nih.gov/pubmed/1951068

5. Kaplan, Rachel, and Stephen Kaplan, *The Experience of Nature: A Psychological Perspective* (Cambridge: Cambridge University Press, 1989).

6. Klepeis, Neil E., "The National Human Activity Pattern Survey (NHAPS): A Resource for Assessing Exposure to Environmental Pollutants," *Journal of Exposure Analysis and Environmental Epidemiology* 11 (2001): 231-52. DOI: 10.1038/Sj.Jea.7500165

7. Louv, Richard, *Last Child in the Woods: Saving Our Children from Nature-Deficit Disorder* (New York: Workman Publishing Company, 2005).

8. Louv, Richard, *Last Child in the Woods: Saving Our Children from Nature-Deficit Disorder* (New York: Workman Publishing Company, 2005).

9. Pergams, O. R. W., and P. A. Zaradic, "Evidence for a Fundamental and Pervasive Shift Away from Nature Based Recreation," *Proceedings*

of the National Academy of Sciences 105 (2007): 2295-300. DOI: 10.1073/Pnas.0709893105

10. Population Reference Bureau, "World Population Highlights 2007: Urbanization," September 2007. http://www.prb.org/publications/data sheets/2007/2007worldpopulationdatasheet.aspx

11. Harvard Medical School, "Newsletter," July 2010, www.health. harvard.edu/newsletters/harvard_health_letter/2010/july

12. Rideout, V. J., U. G. Foehr, and D. F. Roberts, "Generation M2: Media in the Lives of 8 to 18-Year Olds," *The Henry J Kaiser Family Foundation Report*, January 20, 2010. http://www.kff.org/entmedia/8010.cfm

13. Juster, F. T., F. Stafford, and H. Ono, *Changing Times of American Youth: 1981-2003*, Institute for Social Research, Ann Arbor, MI: University of Michigan, www.ns.umich.edu/releases/2004/nov04/teen_time_report.pdf

14. Doheny, Kathleen, "It's Never Too Early to Teach Kids the Activity Habit," *HealthDay*, November 25, 2004.

15. Pretty, J., "The Mental and Physical Health Outcomes of Green Exercise," *International Journal of Environmental Health Research* 15, 5 (October 2005): 319-37.

16. Oppezzo, Marily, "Give Your Ideas Some Legs: The Positive Effect of Walking on Creative Thinking," *Stanford University Journal of Experimental Psychology Learning Memory and Cognition* 40, 4 (July 2014): 1142-52. DOI: 10.1037/A0036577. Epub April 21, 2014

17. Mejia, Robin, "Green Exercise May Be Good for Your Head," *Environmental Science and Technology* 44 (April 21, 2010): 3649. http://pubs.acs.org/doi/full/10.1021/es101129n

18. Godbey, Geoffrey, "Outdoor Recreation, Health, and Wellness; Understanding and Enhancing the Relationship," *Resources for the Future*, May 2009.

19. Ward Thompson, C., J. Roe, P. Aspinall, R. Mitchell, A. Clow, and D. Miller, "More Green Space is Linked to Less Stress in Deprived Communities: Evidence from Salivary Cortisol Patterns," *Landscape and Urban Planning* 105 (2012): 221-29.

20. Jacobs, J. M., "Going Outdoors Daily Predicts Long-term Functional and Health Benefits among Ambulatory Older People," *Journal of Aging and Health* 20, 3 (April 2008): 259-72. DOI: 10.1177/0898264308315427

21. Harvard Medical School, "Newsletter," July 2010. http://www.health.harvard.edu/newsletters/harvard_health_letter/2010/july

22. Ulrich, Roger S., "View Through a Window May Influence Recovery from Surgery," *Science* 224 (April 27, 1984): 420.

23. Russell, Roly, "Humans and Nature: How Knowing and Experiencing Nature Affect Well Being," *Annual Review of Environ-*

ment and Resources 38 (2013): 473. DOI: 10.1146/Annurev_Environ
_012312_110838

24. Stevenson, Robert Louis, *Essay of Travel* (London: Chatto and Windus, 1905).

25. Park, Bum-Jin, "Using Salivary Cortisol and Cerebral Activity as Indicators," *Journal of Physiological Anthropology* 26, 2 (2006): 123-28.

26. Park, Bum-Jin, "Physiological Effects of Shinrin-Yoku (Taking in the Atmosphere of the Forest)—Using Salivary Cortisol and Cerebral Activity as Indicators," *Journal of Physiological Anthropology* 26, 2 (2007): 123-28. DOI: 10.2114/Jpa2.26.123

27. Li, Qing, "Visiting a Forest, But Not a City, Increases Human Natural Killer Activity and Expression of Anticancer Proteins," *International Journal of Immunopathology and Pharmacology* 21, 1 (January-March 2008): 117-27.

28. Kim, W., S. K. Lim, E. J. Chung, and J. M. Woo, "The Effect of Cognitive Behavior Therapy Based Psychotherapy Applied in a Forest Environment on Psychological Changes and Remission of Major Depression," *Psychiatry Investigation* 6 (2009): 245-54.

29. Centers for Disease Control and Prevention, "Key Findings: Trends in the Parent-Report of Health Care Provider-Diagnosis and Medication Treatment for ADHD: United States, 2003-2011," December 2014.

30. Kuo, F., and A. Taylor, "A Potential Natural Treatment for Attention-Deficit/Hyperactivity Disorder: Evidence from a National Study, *American Journal of Public Health* 94, 9 (2004): 1580-86.

31. Schaffer, Linden, "Well on the Road Interview," 2015/2016.

32. Brown, E. T., *Not Without Prejudice: Essays on Assorted Subjects* (Melbourne, Australia: F. W. Cheshire, 1955).

33. Thomson, J. Arthur, "Vis Medicatrix Naturae," Keynote Address at the Annual Meeting of The British Medical Association, 1914.

34. More, T., and B. Payne, "Affective Responses to Natural Areas Near Cities," *Journal of Leisure Research* 10, 1 (1978): 7-12.

35. Aspinall, P., M. Panagiotis, R. Coyne, and J. Roe, "The Urban Brain: Analysing Outdoor Physical Activity with Mobile EEG," *British Journal of Sports Medicine* 6, 3 (2013): 1-7.

36. De Vries, Sjerp, Robert A. Verheij, and Peter P. Groenewegen, "Nature and Health: The Relation Between Health and Green Space in People's Living Environment," paper presented at the Conference Cultural Events and Leisure Systems, Amsterdam, The Netherlands, April 2001.

37. Public Health England, "Ecotherapy: The Green Agenda for Mental Health," (Exec. Summ.) *Mind*, UK. https://www.mind.org.uk/media/273470/ecotherapy.pdf

38. Li, Qing, "Acute Effects of Walking in Forest Environments on Cardiovascular and Metabolic Parameters," *European Journal of Applied Physiology* 111 (2011): 2845-53. DOI: 10.1007/S00421-011-1918-Z

39. Department for Environment, Food & Rural Affairs, "The Natural Choice: Securing the Value of Nature. Presented to Parliament by the Secretary of State for Environment, Food and Rural Affairs, by Command of Her Majesty," United Kingdom, 2011.

40. Shibata, S., and N. Suzuki, "Effects of an Indoor Plant on Creative Task Performance and Mood," *Scandinavian Journal of Psychology* 45 (2004): 373-81.

41. Variety Power of Women Event, 2013. https://www.youtube.com/watch?v=G4Q0oX8wquU

42. McPherson, Miller, et. al., "Social Isolation in America: Changes in Core Discussion Networks Over Two Decades," *American Sociological Review* 71 (June 2006): 353-75.

43. Cacioppo, J. T., and S. Cacioppo, "Social Relationships and Health: The Toxic Effects of Perceived Social Isolation," *Social and Personality Psychology Compass* 8 (2014): 58-72. DOI: 10.1111/Spc3.12087

44. Cacioppo, J. T., "AAAS 2014: Loneliness Is a Major Health Risk for Older Adults," presented in the Science of Resilient Aging at the American Association for the Advancement of Science, February 13-17, 2014.

45. Gammon, Katharine, "Why Loneliness Can Be Deadly," *Livescience*, March 2012, www.livescience.com/18800-loneliness health problems. html

46. Gupta, Sanjay, "Why You Should Treat Loneliness as a Chronic Illness," *Everyday Health*, August 4, 2015.

47. Holt-Lunstad, J., T. B. Smith, and J. B. Layton, "Social Relationships and Mortality Risk: A Meta-Analytic Review," *PLoS Medicine* 7, 7 (2010): E1000316. DOI:10.1371/Journal.Pmed.1000316

48. Cacioppo, J. T., "AAAS 2014: Loneliness Is a Major Health Risk for Older Adults," presented in the Science of Resilient Aging at the American Association for the Advancement of Science, February 13-17, 2014.

49. Holt-Lunstad, J., T. B. Smith, and J. B. Layton, "Social Relationships and Mortality Risk: A Meta-Analytic Review," *PLoS Medicine* 7, 7 (2010): E1000316.

50. Cohen, Sheldon and Ian Brissette, "Social Integration and Health: The Case of the Common Cold," *Journal of Social Structure*, Carnegie Mellon University, Article: Volume 1.

51. Smith, Emily Esfahani, "Social Connection Makes a Better Brain," *The Atlantic*, October 29, 2013.

52. Kross, E., et al., "Facebook Use Predicts Declines in Subjective Well-Being in Young Adults," *PLoS One* 8, 8 (2013): E69841. DOI:10.1371/Journal.Pone.0069841

53. American Public Health Association, "Improving Health and Wellness through Access to Nature," November 5, 2013, Policy Number: 20137.

54. Owens, Judith A., et al., "Impact of Delaying School Start Time on Adolescent Sleep, Mood, and Behavior," *Archives of Pediatrics & Adolescent Medicine* 164, 7 (July 2010): 608-14. DOI:10.1001/Archpediatrics.2010.96

CHAPTER 6

1. Northup, Temple, "Understanding the Relationship between Television Use and Unhealthy Eating: The Mediating Role of Fatalistic Views of Eating Well and Nutritional Knowledge," *The International Journal of Communication and Health* 3 (2014): 10.

2. Dietary Guidelines Advisory Committee, "Scientific Report of 2015," Part A, Executive Summary. https://health.gov/dietaryguidelines/2015-scientific-report/PDFs/02-executive-summary.pdf

3. Carpenter, Kenneth J., "A Short History of Nutritional Science: Part 1 (1785-1885)," *The Journal Of Nutrition* (2003): 638-45.

4. Weil, Andrew, *Natural Health, Natural Medicine* (Boston: Houghton Mifflin Company, 2004), 5.

5. *In Defense of Food*, by Michael Pollan, directed by Michael Schwarz, 2015.

6. American Diabetes Association, "Statistics About Diabetes," April 1, 2016, www.diabetes.org/diabetes-basics/statistics/

7. Boden, Guenther, "Excessive Caloric Intake Acutely Causes Oxidative Stress, GLUT4 Carbonylation, and Insulin Resistance in Healthy Men," *Science Translational Medicine* 7, 304 (September 9, 2015): 304re7. DOI: 10.1126/scitranslmed.aac4765

8. Karl, T., et al., "Y1 Receptors Regulate Aggressive Behavior by Modulating Serotonin Pathways," *Proceedings of the National Academic Sciences of the United States of America* 101, 34 (August 24, 2004): 12742-47.

9. Savage, Stephanie, "Study Finds Warning Signs of Diabetes Can Show Up in Just a Few Days," *ABC Radio*, September 9, 2015.

10. Drake, Victoria, "Inflammation," Linus Pauling Institute. Micronutrient Information Center, Oregon State University, August 2010, http://lpi.oregonstate.edu/mic/micronutrients-health/inflammation

11. Berk, Michael, "So Depression Is an Inflammatory Disease, but Where Does the Inflammation Come From?" *BMC Medicine* (September 2013). DOI: 10.1186/1741-7015-11-200

12. Berk, Michael, "So Depression Is an Inflammatory Disease, but Where Does the Inflammation Come From?" *BMC Medicine* (September 2013).

13. Parvez, S., et al., "Probiotics and Their Fermented Food Products Are Beneficial for Health," *Journal of Applied Microbiology* (April 2006). DOI: 10.1111/J.1365-2672.2006.02963.X

14. Ishige, K., "Flavonoids Protect Neuronal Cells from Oxidative Stress by Three Distinct Mechanisms," *Free Radical Biology and Medicine* 30, 4 (February 15, 2001): 433-46.

15. Konczak, Izabela, "Anthocyanins—More Than Nature's Colours," *Journal of Biomedicine and Biotechnology* 5 (December 1, 2004): 239-40. DOI: 10-1155-S1110724304407013 Pmcid Pmc1082903

16. Rangel-Huerta, O. D., C. M. Aguilera, M. D. Mesa, and A. Gil, "Omega-3 Long Chain Polyunsaturated Fatty Acids Supplementation on Inflammatory Biomakers: A Systematic Review of Randomized Clinical Trials," *British Journal of Nutrition* 107 (2012): 3159-70.

17. Weekes, John, "Mediterranean Diet Could Help Men with Prostate Cancer," *New Zealand Herald*, July 22, 2015.

18. Wu, A. J., "Dietary Omega-3 Fatty Acids Normalize BDNF Levels, Reduce Oxidative Damage, and Counteract Learning Disability after Traumatic Brain Injury in Rats," *Neurotrauma* 21, 10 (October 2004): 1457-67.

19. Lisle, Douglas J., "Break Your Food Addictions," *WebMD*. http://www.webmd.com/food-recipes/features/breaking-food-adictions#1

20. Hyman, Mark, "10 Dramatic Shifts the Occur When You Detox," July 2015. http://drhyman.com/blog/2015/07/03/10-dramatic-shifts-that-occur-when-you-detox/

21. Yamamoto, T., et al., "Effect of Sauna Bathing and Beer Ingestion on Plasma Concentrations of Purine Bases," *Metabolism* 53, 6 (June 2004): 772-76.

22. Nowson, C. A., et al., "Vitamin D and Health in Adults in Australia and New Zealand: A Position Statement," *Medical Journal of Australia* 196, 11 (2012): 686-87.

23. Hansen, Anita L., "Fish Consumption, Sleep, Daily Functioning, and Heart Rate Variability," *American Academy of Sleep Medicine*, University of Bergen, Bergen, Norway, 2014.

24. Mauskop, Alexander and Jasmine Varughese, "Why All Migraine Patients Should be Treated with Magnesium," *Journal of Neural Transmission* 119, 5 (May 2012): 575-79.

25. Planells, E., "Effect of Magnesium Deficiency on Vitamin B2 and B6 Status in the Rat," *Journal of the American College of Nutrition* 16, 4 (August 1997): 352–56.

26. Weil, Andrew, "Vitamin Library," www.drweil.com/drw/u/pag00321/vitamin-library-supplement-facts.html

27. Schaffer, Linden, "Simple Ways to Eat Clean for Overall Wellness," *The Huffington Post Healthy Living*, November 5, 2013.

28. Nielsen, Global Health & Wellness Report, "We Are What We Eat: Healthy Eating Trends Around the World," January 2015. https://www.nielsen.com/content/dam/nielsenglobal/eu/nielseninsights/pdfs/nielsen%20global%20health%20and%20wellness%20report%20-%20january%202015.pdf

29. Dietary Guidelines Advisory Committee, "Scientific Report of 2015," Part A, Executive Summary. https://health.gov/dietaryguidelines/2015-scientific-report/PDFs/02-executive-summary.pdf

30. Brown, Ruth E., et al., "Secular Differences in the Association Between Caloric Intake, Macronutrient Intake, and Physical Activity with Obesity," *Obesity Research Clinical & Practice* 10, 3 (May–June 2016): 243–55. DOI: dx.doi.org/10.1016/j.orcp.2015.08.007

31. Khazan, Olga, "Why It Was Easier to Be Skinny in the 1980s," *The Atlantic*, September 30, 2015.

32. Haiken, Melanie, "The New Theory on Weight Loss: Your Bad Diet Has Damaged Your Brain," *Forbes*, August 21, 2013.

33. Centers for Disease Control and Prevention, "Adult Obesity Facts," September 2015, www.cdc.gov/obesity/data/adult.html.

34. Luppino, F. S., et al., "Overweight, Obesity, and Depression: A Systematic Review and Meta-analysis of Longitudinal Studies," *Archives of General Psychiatry* 67 (2010): 220–29.

35. Fitzpatrick, A. L., et al., "Midlife and Late-Life Obesity and the Risk of Dementia: Cardiovascular Health Study," *Archives of Neurology* 66 (2009): 336–42.

36. Haiken, Melanie, "The New Theory on Weight Loss: Your Bad Diet Has Damaged Your Brain," *Forbes*, August 2013.

37. Nielsen, Global Health & Wellness Report, "We Are What We Eat, Healthy Eating Trends Around the World," January 2015.

38. Reynolds, Gretchen, "Weighing the Evidence on Exercise," *New York Times Magazine*, April 16, 2010.

39. Farshchi, Hamid R., "Deleterious Effects of Omitting Breakfast on Insulin Sensitivity and Fasting Lipid Profiles in Healthy Lean Women," American Society for Clinical Nutrition. http://ajcn.nutrition.org/content/81/2/388. Abstract

40. Healthday News, "The Weird Reason People Snack More while Watching Action Movies," September 2, 2014. http://news.health.com/2014/09/02/action-packed-tv-a-threat-to-your-waistline/

41. Inniss, A. M., B. L. Rice, and S. M. Smith, "Dietary Support of Extended-Duration Bed Rest Studies," *International Journal of Workplace Health Management* 2006. http://ntrs.nasa.gov/archive/nasa/casi.ntrs.nasa.gov/20060018323.pdf

42. Woolf, Virginia, *A Room of One's Own* (London: Hogarth Press, 1929).

43. Dayton, Tian, "Are You Self Medicating Your Emotional Stress with Food?" *The Huffington Post Healthy Living*, November 17, 2011.

44. Gearhardt, M. S., and N. Ashley, "An Examination of the Food Addiction Construct in Obese Patients with Binge Eating Disorder," *International Journal of Eating Disorders* 45, 5 (July 2012): 657-63.

45. Gold, M. S., K. Frost-Pineda, and W. S. Jacobs, "Overeating, Binge Eating, and Eating Disorders as Addictions," *Psychiatric Annals* 33, 2 (February 2003): 117–22.

46. Avena, N. M., P. Rada, and B. G. Hoebel, "Evidence for Sugar Addiction: Behavioral and Neurochemical Effects of Intermittent, Excessive Sugar Intake," *Neuroscience and Biobehavioral Reviews* 32 (2008): 20–39.

47. Van Dijk, Sheri, *Calming the Emotional Storm: Using Dialectical Behavior Therapy Skills to Manage Your Emotions and Balance Your Life* (Oakland, CA: New Harbinger Publications, 2012).

48. Kulkarni, A. A., "Associations Between Diet Quality and Mental Health in Socially Disadvantaged New Zealand Adolescents," *European Journal of Clinical Nutrition* 69, 1 (January 2015): 7983. DOI: 10.1038/Ejcn.2014.130. Epub July 16, 2014

49. Macht, M., "Immediate Effects of Chocolate on Experimentally Induced Mood States," *Appetite* 49, 3 (November 2007): 667-74. Epub May 23, 2007

50. Freeman, M. P., "Omega-3 Fatty Acids in Major Depressive Disorder," *Journal of Clinical Psychiatry* 70, Suppl 5 (2009): 7-11. DOI: 10.4088/Jcp.8157sul C.02

51. Jacka, F. N., N. Cherbuin, K. J. Anstey, and P. Butterworth, "Dietary Patterns and Depressive Symptoms Over Time: Examining the Relationships with Socioeconomic Position, Health Behaviours and Cardiovascular Risk," *PLoS One* 9, 1 (2014): E87657. DOI:10.1371/Journal.Pone.008765

52. Sarris, Jerome, "Nutrients and Herbal Supplements for Mental Health," *Australian Prescriber* 37 (June 2, 2014): 90-93. http://dx.doi.org/10.18773/austprescr.2014.036

53. Kim, Sangmi, "Eating Patterns and Nutritional Characteristics Associated with Sleep Duration," *Public Health Nutrition* 14, 5 (May 2011): 889–95. Published online October 29, 2010. DOI: 10.1017/S136898001000296X PMCID: PMC3179429 NIHMSID: NIHMS322771

54. *Men in Black*, directed by Barry Sonnenfeld, Columbia Pictures, 1997.

55. *In Defense of Food*, by Michael Pollan, directed by Michael Schwarz, 2015.

56. Seidenberg, Casey, "Why Sugar and Caffeine Only Make Your Teen More Stressed During Cram Sessions," *Washington Post*, March 16, 2016.

57. Queensland University of Technology, "Treating Sugar Addiction Like Drug Abuse," *Science Daily*, April 7, 2016, www.sciencedaily.com/releases/2016/04/160407111828.htm

58. Lenoir, M., F. Serre, L. Cantin, and S. H. Ahmed, "Intense Sweetness Surpasses Cocaine Reward," *PLoS ONE* 2, 8 (2007): E698. DOI:10.1371/Journal.Pone.0000698

59. Shariff, M., et al., "Neuronal Nicotinic Acetylcholine Receptor Modulators Reduce Sugar Intake," *PLoS ONE* 11, 3 (2016): E0150270. DOI:10.1371/Journal.Pone.0150270

60. American Heart Association, "Added Sugars," July 20, 2016, www.heart.org/heartorg/healthyliving/healthyeating/nutrition/added-sugars_ucm_305858_article.jsp#.vyy8paodfbc

61. Cleveland Clinic, "How Much Sugar Are You Eating? (Infographic)," June 2013.

62. Rabin, Roni Caryn, "Placing a Cap on Americans' Consumption of Added Sugar," *New York Times*, November 9, 2015.

63. Union of Concerned Scientists, "Added Sugar on the Nutrition Facts Label: Public Comments to the FDA Show Big Food Is Sour on Science," March 2015, www.ucsusa.org/center-science-and-democracy/added-sugar-nutrition-facts-label#.vld7y9-rsv4

64. Yang, Q., "Added Sugar Intake and Cardiovascular Diseases Mortality among US Adults," *JAMA Internal Medicine* 174, 4 (April 2014): 516–24. DOI: 10.1001/Jamainternmed.2013.13563

65. Shah, Amy, "10 Reasons to Think Twice before Going to the Doctor," *mindbodygreen*, May 2, 2014. http://www.mindbodygreen.com/0-13606/10-reasons-to-think-twice-before-going-to-the-doctor-advice-from-an-md.html

66. World Health Organization, "WHO Calls on Countries to Reduce Sugars Intake among Adults and Children," March 4, 2015.

67. World Health Organization, "WHO Calls on Countries to Reduce Sugars Intake Among Adults and Children," March 4, 2015.

68. Rabin, Roni Caryn, "Placing a Cap on Americans' Consumption of Added Sugar," *New York Times*, November 9, 2015.

69. Ramsey, Lydia, "The USDA Just Released a Massive New Report on What's Actually Healthy," *Business Insider*, January 7, 2016. http://www.businessinsider.com/usda-2015-guidelines-2016-12

70. *Fresh*, directed by Ana Sofia Joanes, Ripple Effect Films, 2009.

71. Moss, Michael, "The Extraordinary Science of Addictive Junk Food," *The New York Times Magazine*, February 2013.

72. *In Defense of Food*, directed by Michael Schwarz, 2015.

73. Sifferlin, Alexandra, "Salt Sugar Fat: Q&A with Author Michael Moss," *Time Magazine*, February 26, 2013.

74. Bengmark, S., "Gut Microbiota, Immune Development and Function," *Pharmacological Research* 69 (2013): 87–113.

75. Berk, Michael, "So Depression Is an Inflammatory Disease, But Where Does the Inflammation Come From?" *BMC Medicine*, September 2013. DOI:10.1186/1741 7015 11 200)

76. Nielsen, Global Health & Wellness Report, "We Are What We Eat: Healthy Eating Trends around the World," January 2015. https://www.nielsen.com/content/dam/nielsenglobal/eu/nielseninsights/pdfs/nielsen%20global%20health%20and%20wellness%20report%20 %20january%202015.pdf

77. Nielsen, Global Health & Wellness Report, "We Are What We Eat: Healthy Eating Trends around the World," January 2015.

78. Nielsen, Global Health & Wellness Report, "We Are What We Eat: Healthy Eating Trends around the World," January 2015.

79. *In Defense of Food*, directed by Michael Schwarz, 2015.

80. Sifferlin, Alexandra, "Salt Sugar Fat: Q&A with Author Michael Moss," *Time Magazine*, February 26, 2013.

81. Hair, Marilyn and Jon Sharpe, "Fast Facts about the Human Microbiome," The Center for Ecogenetics and Environmental Health, University of Washington, January 2014.

82. Brown, Alan Kavli Foundation, "Microbial Manifesto: The Global Push to Understand the Microbiome," *Google Hangout* session, March 2, 2016, transcribed at http://www.livescience.com/53916-understanding-life-means-understanding-microbes.html

83. Hair, Marilyn and Jon Sharpe, "Fast Facts about the Human Microbiome," The Center for Ecogenetics and Environmental Health, University of Washington, January 2014.

84. Hair, Marilyn and Jon Sharpe, "Fast Facts about the Human Microbiome," The Center for Ecogenetics and Environmental Health, University of Washington, January 2014.

85. Gibson, G. R., H. M. Probert, J. Van Loo, R. A. Rastall, and M. B. Roberfroid, "Dietary Modulation of the Human Colonic Microbiota: Updating the Concept of Prebiotics," *Nutrition Research Reviews* 17, 2 (2004): 259-75.

86. Kotzampassi, K., and E. J. Giamarellos-Bourboulis, "Probiotics for Infectious Diseases: More Drugs, Less Dietary Supplementation," *International Journal of Antimicrobial Agents* 40 (2012): 288-96.

87. Bengmark, S., "Gut Microbiota, Immune Development and Function," *Pharmacological Research* 69 (2013): 87-113.

88. Hildebrandt, M. A., et al., "High Fat Diet Determines the Composition of the Murine Gut Microbiome Independently of Obesity," *Gastroenterology* 137, 5 (2009): 1716-24.

89. Arora, Tulika, "Probiotics: Interaction with Gut Microbiome and Antiobesity Potential," *Nutrition Journal* 29, 4 (April 2002): 591. DOI: http://dx.doi.org/10.1016/j.nut.2012.07.017

90. Proal, A. D., P. J. Albert, and T. G. Marshall, "The Human Microbiome and Autoimmunity," *Current Opinion in Rheumatology* 25, 2 (March 2013): 234-40. DOI: 10.1097/BOR.0b013e32835cedbf

91. Morning Edition, NPR, "Gut Bacteria Might Guide the Workings of Our Minds," November 18, 2013. http://www.npr.org/sections/health-shots/2013/11/18/244526773/gut-bacteria-might-guide-the-workings-of-our-minds

92. Collins, Stephen M., "The Adoptive Transfer of Behavioral Phenotype via the Intestinal Microbiota: Experimental Evidence and Clinical Implications," *Ecology and Industrial Microbiology*, Special Section: Innate Immunity, 16, 3 (June 2013): 240-45.

93. Weil, Andrew, *Natural Health, Natural Medicine* (Boston: Houghton Mifflin Company, 2004).

94. Dietary Guidelines Advisory Committee, "Scientific Report of 2015," Part A, Executive Summary. https://health.gov/dietaryguidelines/2015-scientific-report/PDFs/02-executive-summary.pdf

95. Northup, Temple, "Understanding the Relationship between Television Use and Unhealthy Eating: The Mediating Role of Fatalistic Views of Eating Well and Nutritional Knowledge," *The International Journal of Communication and Health* 3 (2014): 10.

96. Northup, Temple, "Understanding the Relationship between Television Use and Unhealthy Eating: The Mediating Role of Fatalistic Views of Eating Well and Nutritional Knowledge," *The International Journal of Communication and Health* 3 (2014): 10.

97. Horovitz, Bruce, "Younger Folks Want Healthier Food—And Will Pay for It," *USA Today*, January 19, 2015.

98. Sifferlin, Alexandra, "Salt Sugar Fat: Q&A with Author Michael Moss," *Time Magazine*, February 26, 2013.

99. *In Defense of Food*, directed by Michael Schwarz, 2015.
100. University of Liverpool, "Fish Oil May Stall Effects of Junk Food on Brain," *Science Daily*, May 14, 2013, www.sciencedaily.com/releases/2013/05/130514101455.htm

CHAPTER 7

1. Twain, Mark, *The Innocents Abroad* (Hartford, CT: American Publishing Company, 1869), 243.
2. US Travel Association, "Travel Effect Report," 2013.
3. US Travel Association, "Travel Effect Report," 2013.
4. US Travel Association, "Travel Effect Report," 2013.
5. Project: Time Off, "The Role of Business Travel in the U.S. Economy," 2013.
6. Global Business Travel Association, "U.S. Business Travel Marketplace to Remain Stable and Steady Despite Sea of Global Volatility," January 12, 2016.
7. US Travel Association, "Travel Effect Report," 2013.
8. Rapoza, Kenneth, "Business Travel Market to Surpass $1 Trillion This Year," *Forbes*, August 6, 2013.
9. Bell, Katie Kelly, "What Today's Business Traveler Wants: Ten Findings from Virgin Atlantic," *Forbes*, October 20, 2014.
10. Richards, Catherine, "Business Travel and Self-Rated Health, Obesity, and Cardiovascular Disease Risk Factors," *Journal of Occupational & Environmental Medicine* 53, 4 (April 2011): 358–63. DOI: 10.1097/Jom.0b013e3182143e77
11. Statista, "Statistics and Facts on the Global Business Travel Industry," 2014. http://www.statista.com/topics/2439/global-business-travel-industry/
12. Peltier, Dan, "Business Travelers Unsure If 'Bleisure' Travel Is Allowed, but Doing It Anyway," *Skift*, October 22, 2014. https://skift.com/2014/10/22/business-travelers-unsure-if-bleisure-travel-is-allowed-but-doing-it-anyway/
13. Balakrishnan, Anita, "Uber, Start-ups Shake Up Business," *CNBC*, January 2016. http://www.cnbc.com/2016/01/21/uber-start-ups-shake-up-business-travel.html
14. Baskas, Harriet, "JetBlue Sprouts a Potato Farm at New York JFK," Special for *USA Today*, October 2015.
15. Baskas, Harriet, "JetBlue Sprouts a Potato Farm at New York JFK," Special for *USA Today*, October 2015.
16. Baskas, Harriet, "JetBlue Sprouts a Potato Farm at New York JFK," Special for *USA Today*, October 2015.

17. Karmin, Craig, "Equinox Fitness Clubs Expand to Hotels," *The Wall Street Journal*, April 2015.

18. Schaffer, Linden, "Well on the Road Interview," 2015/2016.

19. US Travel Association, "Travel Effect Report," 2013.

20. Chalmer, William, "America's Vacation Deficit Disorder," *The Huffington Post*, July 29, 2012.

21. Ali, Rafat, "Travel Habits of Americans: 42 Percent Didn't Take Any Vacation Days in 2014," *Skift*, January 5, 2015. https://skift.com/2015/01/05/travel-habits-of-americans-41-percent-didnt-take-any-vacation-days-in-2014/

22. Expedia, "2015 Vacation Deprivation Study: Europe Leads World in Paid Vacation Time While Americans and Asians Lag," November 26, 2015.

23. Nawijn, Jeroen, et al., "Vacationers Happier, but Most Not Happier After a Holiday," *Applied Research Quality Life* 5 (February 2010): 35–47. DOI: 10.1007/S11482-009-9091-9

24. US Travel Association, "US Travel Answer Sheet," 2015. https://www.ustravel.org/sites/default/files/media%20root/document/us_travel_answersheet_dec2015_final%20(2).pdf

25. Belsky, Gary and Tom Gilovich, "Want Happiness? Don't Buy More Stuff—Go on Vacation," *Time Magazine*, July 21, 2011.

26. Project: Time Off, "The Work Martyr's Children: How Kids Are Harmed by America's Lost Week," September 2015. http://www.project-timeoff.com/sites/default/files/PTO_WMC_Report.pdf

27. Project: Time Off, "The Work Martyr's Children: How Kids Are Harmed by America's Lost Week," September 2015.

28. Ray, Rebecca, Milla Sanes, and John Schmitt, "No-Vacation Nation Revisited," Center for Economic and Policy Research, May 2013. http://cepr.net/publications/reports/no-vacation-nation-2013

29. Federal Deposit Insurance Corporation, "Vacation Policies FIL-52-95," August 3, 1995.

30. Society for Human Resources Management, "Vacation's Impact on the Workplace Survey," August 22–September 5, 2013. https://www.shrm.org/hr-today/trends-and-forecasting/research-and-surveys/pages/shrm-us-travel-vacation-benefits.aspx

31. Project: Time Off, "The Role of Business Travel in the U.S. Economy," 2013.

32. Project: Time Off, "The Role of Business Travel in the U.S. Economy," 2013.

33. Project: Time Off, "The Hidden Costs of Unused Leave," Oxford Economics Study, 2015.

34. Glassdoor Employment Confidence Survey, "Average U.S. Employee Only Takes Half of Earned Vacation Time," April 3, 2014.

35. Crane, Brent, "For a More Creative Brain, Travel," *The Atlantic*, March 31, 2015.

36. Branson, Richard, "How to Take an Inspiration Vacation," *Entrepreneur Magazine*, September 2013.

37. Galinsky, Adam D., "Fashion With a Foreign Flair: Professional Experiences Abroad Facilitate the Creative Innovations of Organizations," *Academy of Management Journal* 58, 1 (May 2014): 195-220.

38. Westman, M., and D. Etzion, "The Impact of Vacation and Job Stress on Burnout and Absenteeism," *Psychology and Health* 16, 5 (2001): 595-606.

39. Mintel, "Voyage of Discovery as Education Becomes Latest Travel Trend," September 11, 2009. http://www.mintel.com/press-centre/travel/voyage-of-discovery-as-education-becomes-latest-travel-trend

40. De Bloom, Jessica, et al., "Vacation (After-) Effects on Employee Health and Well-Being and the Role of Vacation Activities, Experiences and Sleep," *Journal of Happiness*, May 2012. DOI: 10.1007/S10902-012-9345-3

41. Taris, Toon W., "Investigating the Associations among Overtime Work, Health Behaviors, and Health: A Longitudinal Study among Full-Time Employees," *International Journal of Behavioral Medicine* 18 (2011): 352-60. DOI: 10.1007/S12529-010-9103-7.

42. Thaik M. D., Cynthia M., "Take a Vacation for Your Health," *Psychology Today*, May 2013. https://www.psychologytoday.com/blog/the-heart/201305/take-vacation-your-health

43. Gump, B., and K. Matthews, "Are Vacations Good for Your Health? The 9-Year Mortality Experience After the Multiple Risk Factor Intervention Trial," *Psychosomatic Medicine* 62, 5 (2000): 608-12.

44. Chikani, Vatsal, "Vacations Improve Mental Health among Rural Women," *Wisconsin Medical Journal* 104, 6 (2005): 20-23.

45. Nawijn, Jeroen, et al., "Vacationers Happier, But Most Not Happier After a Holiday," *Applied Research Quality Life* 5 (February 2010): 35-47.

46. Borins, M., *Go Away: Just for the Health of It*, (Downsview, ON: Wholistic Press, 2000).

47. Yesawich, Peter C., "National Travel Monitor: Travelers Trading Down, Not Out," *Hotel & Motel Management* 224, 10 (January 9, 2009): 20.

48. Zimmermann, Julia and Franz J. Neyer, "Do We Become a Different Person When Hitting the Road? Personality Development of Sojourners," *Journal of Personality and Social Psychology* 105, 3 (Sep-

tember 2013): 515-30. http://psycnet.apa.org/?&fa=main.doilanding&doi=10.1037/a0033019

49. Cralle, Trevor, *Flinging Monkeys at the Coconuts: A Traveler's Companion of Quotations* (New York: Ten Speed Press, 1993).

50. Mayerowitz, Scott, "How to Beat Jet Lag," *Travel and Leisure Magazine*, August 2015, www.travelandleisure.com/articles/how-to-beat-jet-lag

51. Rosenbloom, Stephanie, "A Battle Plan for Jet Lag," *The New York Times*, August 15, 2012.

52. Stevens, Richard, "The Key to Feeling Well Rested Isn't Just the Amount of Time You Sleep," *Business Insider*, April 6, 2015.

53. Fuller, Patrick M., Jun Lu, and Clifford B. Saper, "Differential Rescue of Light- and Food-Entrainable Circadian Rhythms," *Science* 320, 5879 (May 23, 2008): 1074-77. DOI: 10.1126/Science.1153277

54. Fuller, Patrick M., Jun Lu, and Clifford B. Saper, "Differential Rescue of Light- and Food-Entrainable Circadian Rhythms," *Science* 320, 5879 (May 23, 2008): 1074-77.

55. Seneca, Lucius Annaeus, "Letter LXXXIV: On Gathering Ideas, Line 13—*Epistulae Morales ad Lucilium*" (Moral Letters to Lucilius).

56. Global Wellness Institute, "Global Spa & Wellness Economy Monitor," January 2015.

57. Global Wellness Institute, "Global Spa & Wellness Economy Monitor," January 2015.

58. Fielding, Thomas (John Wade), *Select Proverbs of All Nations* (1824), 216.

59. Sherwood, Lauralee, *Human Physiology: From Cells to Systems*, Ninth Edition (Independence, KY: Cengage Learning, 2016).

60. Liu, Bor-Shong, and Chia-Chen Wu, "Survey of Health Problems for Long-Haul Flight Travelers," Department of Industrial Engineering and Management, St. John's University. Project No. Nsc 98-2221-E-129-003.

61. Ruppel, Glenn, Jim Avila, and Mark Greenblat, "Mice, Roaches Seen by FDA Inspecting Airline Food," *ABC News*, November 2012.

CHAPTER 8

1. Nesse, Randolph, and George Williams, *Why We Get Sick: The New Science of Darwinian Medicine* (New York: First Vintage Books, 1996).

2. Bailey, Sarah, "Gwyneth Unveiled," *Harper's Bazaar*, April 2013.

3. Merriam-Webster, "Intuition." http://www.merriam-webster.com/dictionary/intuition

4. Hanh, Thich Nhat, *Cultivating the Mind of Love* (Berkeley, CA: Parallax Press, 1996).

5. Rock, David and Jeffrey Schwartz, "The Neuroscience of Leadership," *Summer Strategy + Business*, 43, May 30, 2006. http://www.strategy-business.com/article/06207?gko=6da0a

6. Rock, David and Jeffrey Schwartz, "The Neuroscience of Leadership," *Summer Strategy + Business*, 43, May 30, 2006.

7. Plutchik, Michael, and Henry Kellerman, eds., *Biological Foundations of Emotion* (Cambridge, MA: Academic Press, 1986).

8. Rock, David and Jeffrey Schwartz, "The Neuroscience of Leadership," *Summer Strategy + Business*, 43, May 30, 2006.

9. Rock, David and Jeffrey Schwartz, "The Neuroscience of Leadership," *Summer Strategy + Business*, 43, May 30, 2006.

10. Vickery, Donald, Larry Matson, and Carol Vickery, *Live Young, Think Young, Be Young* (Boulder, CO: Bull Publishing Company, 2012).

11. Perlow, Leslie A., "Overcome Your Work Addiction," *Harvard Business Review*, May 2, 2012. https://hbr.org/2012/05/overcome-your-work-addiction.html

12. Bernstein, Gabrielle, "The Spiritual Secret to Success," July 2015. http://gabbyb.tv/blogs/the-spiritual-secret-to-success

13. Hines, Ree, "Oprah Unveils Her Weight-Loss Transformation, Talks 'Best Body' in O," *Today*, March 11, 2016.

14. Dell, Michael S., "Commencement Address 2003," 2003, www.utexas.edu/commencement/2003/spring/speech.html

15. Fredrickson, Barbara L., et al., "Open Hearts Build Lives: Positive Emotions, Induced Through Loving-Kindness Meditation, Build Consequential Personal Resources," *The Journal of Personality and Social Psychology* 95, 5 (November 2008): 1045–62. DOI: 10.1037/A0013262

16. Cuddy, Amy, J. C., Caroline A. Wilmuth, and Dana R. Carney, "The Benefit of Power Posing Before a High-Stakes Social Evaluation," *Harvard Business School*, Working Paper, No. 13-027, September 2012.

17. Cuddy, Amy, J. C., Caroline A. Wilmuth, and Dana R. Carney, "The Benefit of Power Posing Before a High-Stakes Social Evaluation," *Harvard Business School*, Working Paper, No. 13-027, September 2012.

18. Kasem, Casey, "Casey Kasem's Final American Top 20 Broadcast," July 2009. https://www.youtube.com/watch?v=lCxq6vjAvWs

19. McClelland, David C., *Human Motivation* (Cambridge: Cambridge University Press, 1987).

20. Michigan State University, "Virtual Workout Partners Spur Better Results, Study Finds," *ScienceDaily*, www.sciencedaily.com/releases/2011/05/110518161707.htm

BIBLIOGRAPHY

101st Congress (1989–1990). "H.R.3562—Nutrition Labeling and Education Act of 1990." House—Energy and Commerce. 11/8/1990 Became Public Law No: 101-535.

60 Minutes with Anderson Cooper. "Mindfulness." December 14, 2014. http://www. cbsnews.com/news/mindfulness-anderson-cooper-60-minutes/

Acquity Group. "2014 State of the Internet of Things Study." Acquity Group. http:// www.acquitygroup.com/news-andideas/thought-leadership/article/detail/acquity-group-2014-internet-of-things-study

Action on Sugar. "Shocking Amount of Sugar Found in Many Hot Flavoured Drinks." February 17, 2016. www.actiononsugar.org/news%20ccntrc/surveys%20 /2016/170865.html#sthash.5fr3he4u.dpuf

Afonso, R. F. "Yoga Decreases Insomnia in Postmenopausal Women: A Randomized Clinical Trial." *Menopause*, February 2012; 19(2): 186–93. DOI: 10.1097/Gme .0b013e318228225f

Agnew, Harriett. "'Mindfulness' Gives Stressed-Out Bankers Something to Think About." *London Financial Times*, May 4, 2014.

Akerstedt, T., et al. "Awakening from Sleep." *Sleep Medicine Reviews*, 2002; 6(4). https:// www.ncbi.nlm.nih.gov/pubmed/12531132

Ali, Rafat. "Travel Habits of Americans: 42 Percent Didn't Take Any Vacation Days in 2014." *Skift*, January 5, 2015. https://skift.com/2015/01/05/travel-habits-of-americans-41-percent-didnt-take-any-vacation-days-in-2014/

Altena, Ellemarije, et al. "Reduced Orbitofrontal and Parietal Gray Matter in Chronic Insomnia: A Voxel-Based Morphometric Study." *Biological Psychiatry Journal*, September 2009; 67(2). DOI: http://dx.doi.org/10.1016/j.biopsych.2009.08.003

American Academy of Neurology. "Hold the Diet Soda? Sweetened Drinks Linked to Depression, Coffee Tied to Lower Risk." January 8, 2013. https://www.aan.com/ pressroom/home/pressrelease/1128

American Diabetes Association. "Statistics About Diabetes." April 1, 2016. http://www.diabetes.org/diabetes-basics/statistics/

American Heart Association. "Added Sugars." July 20, 2016. http://www.heart.org/heartorg/healthyliving/healthyeating/nutrition/added-sugars_ucm_305858_article.jsp#.vyy8paodfbc

American Heart Association. "Trans Fats." October 2015. http://www.heart.org/heartorg/healthyliving/fatsandoils/fats101/trans-fats_ucm_301120_article.jsp#.vyy_saodfbc

American Institute of Stress. "Workplace Stress." http://www.cdc.gov/niosh/pdfs/87-111.pdf

American Psychological Association. "Stress in America: Our Health at Risk." January 11, 2012. https://www.apa.org/news/press/releases/stress/2011/final-2011.pdf

American Psychological Association. "Stress in America: Are Teens Adopting Adults' Stress Habits?" 2014. https://www.apa.org/news/press/releases/stress/2013/stress-report.pdf

American Public Health Association. "Improving Health and Wellness through Access to Nature." November 5, 2013, Policy Number: 20137.

Anwar, Yasmin. "Sleep Loss Linked to Psychiatric Disorders." *UC Berkeley*, October 22, 2015. http://www.berkeley.edu/news/media/releases/2007/10/22_sleeploss.shtml

Anxiety and Depression Association of America. "Exercise for Stress and Anxiety." July 2014. http://www.adaa.org/living-with-anxiety/managing-anxiety/exercise-stress-and-anxiety

Arora, Tulika. "Probiotics: Interaction with Gut Microbiome and Antiobesity Potential." *Nutrition Journal*, April 2002; 29(4): 591. DOI: http://Dx.Doi.Org/10.1016/J.Nut.2012.07.017

Aspinall, P., M. Panagiotis, R. Coyne, and J. Roe. "The Urban Brain: Analysing Outdoor Physical Activity with Mobile EEG." *British Journal of Sports Medicine*, 2013; 6(3): 1–7.

Avena, N. M., P. Rada, and B. G. Hoebel. "Evidence for Sugar Addiction: Behavioral and Neurochemical Effects of Intermittent, Excessive Sugar Intake." *Neuroscience and Biobehavioral Reviews*, 2008; 32: 20–39.

Bai, Yang, et al. "Comparison of Different Activity Monitors." *Medicine and Science in Sports & Exercise*, August 2015.

Bailey, Sarah. "Gwyneth Unveiled." *Harper's Bazaar*, April 2013.

Balakrishnan, Anita. "Uber, Start-Ups Shake Up Business." *CNBC*, January 2016. http://www.cnbc.com/2016/01/21/uber-start-ups-shake-up-business-travel.html

Balasubramaniam, M., S. Telles, and P. M. Doraiswamy. "Yoga on Our Minds: A Systematic Review of Yoga for Neuropsychiatric Disorders." *Frontiers in Psychiatry*, 2013; 3: 117. DOI: 10.3389/Fpsyt.2012.00117

Baldauf, Sarah. "From 4 Long-lived Cultures, 9 Tips For Longevity." *U.S. News & World Report*, March 25, 2008. http://health.usnews.com/health-news/family-health/articles/2008/03/25/from-4-long-lived-cultures-9-tips-for-longevity

Barnes, Christopher M. "Sleep-deprived People Are More Likely to Cheat." *Harvard Business Review*, May 31, 2013.

Baskas, Harriet. "JetBlue Sprouts a Potato Farm at New York JFK." Special for *USA Today*, October 2015.

Basner, Mathias, et al. "Sociodemographic Characteristics and Waking Activities and Their Role in the Timing and Duration of Sleep." *Sleep*, 2014; 37(12). http://dx.doi.org/10.5665/sleep.4238

Becker, Gay. "Self-Care among Chronically Ill African Americans: Culture, Health Disparities, and Health Insurance Status." *American Journal for Public Health*, 2003; 94(12): 2066–73.

Belenky, G. "Patterns of Performance Degradation and Restoration During Sleep Restriction and Subsequent Recovery: A Sleep Dose Response Study." *Journal of Sleep Research*, March 2003; 12: 1–12.

Bell, Katie Kelly. "What Today's Business Traveler Wants: Ten Findings from Virgin Atlantic." *Forbes*, October 20, 2014.

Belsky, Gary and Tom Gilovich. "Want Happiness? Don't Buy More Stuff—Go on Vacation." *Time Magazine*, July 21, 2011.

Bengmark, S. "Gut Microbiota, Immune Development and Function." *Pharmacological Research*, 2013; 69: 87–113.

Berk, Michael. "So Depression Is an Inflammatory Disease, but Where Does the Inflammation Come From?" *BMC Medicine*, September 2013. DOI: 10.1186/1741_7015_11_200

Bernstein, Gabrielle. "The Spiritual Secret to Success." July 2015. http://Gabbyb.Tv/Blogs/The-Spiritual-Secret-To-Success

Berry, Leonard, Ann Mirabito, and William Baun. "What's the Hard Return on Employee Wellness Programs?" *Harvard Business Review*, December 2010. https://hbr.org/2010/12/whats-the-hard-return-on-employee-wellness-programs

Bidwell, Allie. "Study: Physical Fitness Linked to Brain Fitness." *U.S. News & World Report*, August 19, 2014.

Blanaru, Monica. "The Effects of Music Relaxation and Muscle Relaxation Techniques on Sleep Quality and Emotional Measures among Individuals with Posttraumatic Stress Disorder." *Mental Illness Journal*, July 26, 2012; 4(2): E13.

Blanding, Michael. "National Health Costs Could Decrease If Managers Reduce Work Stress." *Harvard Business School*, January 26, 2015. http://hbswk.hbs.edu/item/7491.html

Blask, David, et al. "Light Pollution: Adverse Health Effects of Nighttime Lighting." Action of the AMA House of Delegates 2012 Annual Meeting: Council on Science and Public Health Report 4. http://www.atmob.org/library/resources/ama%20health%20effects%20light%20at%20night.pdf

Blue Zones. "Our Approach." https://www.bluezones.com/services/our-approach

Boden, Guenther. "Excessive Caloric Intake Acutely Causes Oxidative Stress, GLUT4 Carbonylation, and Insulin Resistance in Healthy Men." *Science Transla-*

tional Medicine, September 9, 2015; 7(304): 304re7. DOI: 10.1126/scitranslmed. aac4765

Booth, Frank W. "Lack of Exercise Is a Major Cause of Chronic Diseases." *Comprehensive Physiology*, April 2012; 2(2): 1143–211. DOI: 10.1002/Cphy.C110025, Pmcid: Pmc4241367, Nihmsid: Nihms603913

Borins, M. *Go Away: Just for the Health of It*. Downsview, ON: Wholistic Press, 2000.

Borzykowski, Bryan. "Successful Executives and the Four-hour Sleep Myth." *Harvard Business Review*, October 12, 2012. https://hbr.org/2012/10/if-youre-too-busy-to-meditate.html

Branson, Richard. "How to Take an Inspiration Vacation." *Entrepreneur Magazine*, September 2013.

Bregman, Peter. "If You're Too Busy to Meditate, Read This." *Harvard Business Review*, October 2012.

Brendel, David. "There Are Risks to Mindfulness at Work." *Harvard Business Review*, February 11, 2015. https://hbr.org/2015/02/there-are-risks-to-mindfulness-at-work

Brewer, J. A. "Mindfulness Training for Smoking Cessation: Results from a Randomized Controlled Trial." *Drug and Alcohol Dependence*, December 1, 2011; 119(1–2): 72–80. DOI: 10.1016/J.Drugalcdep.2011.05.027. Epub July 1, 2011.

Brewer, Judson. "Meditation Experience Is Associated with Differences in Default Mode Network Activity and Connectivity." *Proceedings of the National Academy of Sciences of the United States of America*, December 13, 2011; 108(50): 20254–59. DOI: 10.1073/Pnas.1112029108. Epub November 23, 2011.

Bromanfulks, J. J. "Effects of Aerobic Exercise on Anxiety Sensitivity." *Behaviour Research and Therapy*, 2004; 42(2); 125–36.

Brooks, Arthur C. "Rising to Your Level of Misery at Work." *New York Times*, September 5, 2015.

Brown, Alan. "Microbial Manifesto: The Global Push to Understand the Microbiome." *Google Hangout Session*, March 2, 2016, transcribed at http://www.livescience.com/53916-understanding-life-means-understanding-microbes.html

Brown, E. T. *Not Without Prejudice: Essays on Assorted Subjects*. Melbourne, Australia: F. W. Cheshire, 1955.

Brown, Ruth E., et al. "Secular Differences in the Association Between Caloric Intake, Macronutrient Intake, and Physical Activity with Obesity." *Obesity Research Clinical & Practice*, May–June 2016; 10(3): 243–55. DOI: dx.doi.org/10.1016/j.orcp.2015.08.007

Buettner, Dan, *The Blue Zones: Lessons for Living Longer from the People Who've Lived the Longest*. Washington, DC: National Geographic Society, 2008.

Burton, Katherine, "To Make a Killing on Wall Street, Start Meditating." *Bloomberg Business*, May 27, 2014.

Cacioppo, J. T. "AAAS 2014: Loneliness Is a Major Health Risk for Older Adults." Presented in the Science of Resilient Aging at the American Association for the Advancement of Science, February 13–17, 2014.

Cacioppo, J. T., and S. Cacioppo. "Social Relationships and Health: The Toxic Effects of Perceived Social Isolation." *Social and Personality Psychology Compass*, 2014; 8: 58–72. DOI: 10.1111/Spc3.12087

Careerbuilder Survey. "Teachers, Engineers and Scientists among Most Likely to Gain Weight on the Job." May 2013. Conducted online within the U.S. by Harris Interactive. http://www.careerbuilder.com/share/aboutus/pressreleasesdetail.aspx?sd=5/30/2013&id=pr760&ed=12/31/2013

Carlson, Emily. "Resetting Our Clocks: New Details about How the Body Tells Time." *NIH—National Institute of General Medical Sciences*, March 2014.

Carlson, Linda E., et al. "Mindfulness-Based Cancer Recovery and Supportive-Expressive Therapy Maintain Telomere Length Relative to Controls in Distressed Breast Cancer Survivors." *Cancer*, November 2014; 12(2): 21–25. DOI: 10.1002/Cncr.29063

Carpenter, Kenneth J. "A Short History of Nutritional Science: Part 1 (1785–1885)." *The Journal of Nutrition*, 2003; 638–45.

CBS This Morning. "Aetna CEO Mark Bertolini on Changing Workplace and Health Care." March 26, 2015. http://www.cbsnews.com/videos/aetna-ceo-mark-bertolini-on-changing-workplace-and-health-care/

Centers for Disease Control and Prevention. "Adult Obesity Facts." September 2015. www.cdc.gov/obesity/data/adult.html

Centers for Disease Control and Prevention. "Behavioral Risk Factor Surveillance Survey 2008–2009." www.cdc.gov/BRFSS

Centers for Disease Control and Prevention. "Chronic Diseases: The Power to Prevent, the Call to Control: At a Glance 2009." 2009.

Centers for Disease Control and Prevention. "Heart Disease Fact Sheet." November 30, 2015.

Centers for Disease Control and Prevention. "Key Findings: Trends in the Parent-Report of Health Care Provider-Diagnosis and Medication Treatment for ADHD: United States, 2003–2011." December 2014.

Centers for Disease Control and Prevention. "Physical Activity—Glossary of Terms." June 2015.

Centers for Disease Control and Prevention. "Short Sleep Duration among Workers—United States, 2010." *Morbidity and Mortality Weekly Report*, April 27, 2012; 61(16): 281–85.

Centers for Disease Control and Prevention. "Stress at Work." National Institute of Occupational Safety and Health, 2014. www.cdc.gov/niosh/docs/99-101/

Chalmer, William. "America's Vacation Deficit Disorder." *The Huffington Post*, July 29, 2012.

Chang, Anne-Marie. "Evening Use of Light-Emitting Ereaders Negatively Affects Sleep, Circadian Timing, and Next-Morning Alertness." National Institutes of Health, Brigham and Women's Hospital, January 27, 2015.

Chevalier, Gaetan, et al. "Earthing: Health Implications of Reconnecting the Human Body to the Earth's Surface Electrons." *Journal of Environmental and Public Health*, 2012; Article ID 291541. http://dx.doi.org/10.1155/2012/291541

Chikani, Vatsal. "Vacations Improve Mental Health among Rural Women." *Wisconsin Medical Journal*, 2005; 104(6): 20–23.

Chopra, Deepak. "Why Wall Streeters Need to Meditate." *CNBC*, March 2015.

Chrysohoou, C. "High Intensity, Interval Exercise Improves Quality of Life of Patients with Chronic Heart Failure: A Randomized Controlled Trial." *The Quaterly Journal of Medicine*, 2014; 107: 25–32. DOI: 10.1093/qjmed/hct194. Advance Access Publication September 30, 2013.

Cleveland Clinic. "How Much Sugar Are You Eating? (Infographic)." June 2013.

Cohen, Sheldon and Ian Brissette. "Social Integration and Health: The Case of the Common Cold." *Journal of Social Structure*, Article: Volume 1. Carnegie Mellon University.

Collins, Stephen M. "The Adoptive Transfer of Behavioral Phenotype Via the Intestinal Microbiota: Experimental Evidence and Clinical Implications." *Ecology and Industrial Microbiology*, Special Section: Innate Immunity, June 2013; 16(3): 240–45.

Colwell, Christopher. "Eating During Sleep Periods May Impair Memory." Presented at Neuroscience 2014, the Annual Meeting of the Society for Neuroscience.

Colzato, Lorenza. "Meditate to Create: The Impact of Focused-Attention and Open-Monitoring Training on Convergent and Divergent Thinking." *Institute for Psychological Research*, Leiden University (2012).

The Commonwealth Fund. "National Trend in the Cost of Employer Health Insurance Coverage." 2003–2013. http://www.commonwealthfund.org/~/media/files/publications/issue-brief/2014/dec/1793_collins_nat_premium_trends_2003_2013.pdf

Confino, J. O. "Thich Nhat Hanh: Is Mindfulness Being Corrupted by Business and Finance?" *The Guardian*, March 28, 2014.

Corporate Leadership Council. "Driving Performance and Retention Through Employee Engagement." 2004. http://www.usc.edu/programs/cwfl/assets/pdf/employee%20engagement.pdf

Coulson, J. C., J. McKenna, and M. Field. "Exercising at Work and Self-Reported Work Performance." *International Journal of Workplace Health Management*, 2008; 1(3): 176–97.

Cralle, Trevor. *Flinging Monkeys at the Coconuts: A Traveler's Companion of Quotations*. New York: Ten Speed Press, 1993.

Crane, Brent. "For a More Creative Brain, Travel." *The Atlantic*, March 31, 2015.

Cuddy, Amy, J. C., Caroline A. Wilmuth, and Dana R. Carney. "The Benefit of Power Posing Before a High-Stakes Social Evaluation." *Harvard Business School*, Working Paper, No. 13-027. September 2012.

Cutrone, Carolyn and Max Nisen. "19 Successful People Who Barely Sleep." *Business Insider*, September 2012.

Czeisler, Charles. "A Sleep Epidemic." *TED Talk*, 2001. www.youtube.com/watch?v=p4UxLpoNCxU

Davidson, Richard J. "Buddha's Brain: Neuroplasticity and Meditation." *IEEE Signal Processing Magazine*, January 1, 2008; 25(1): 176-74. www.ncbi.nlm.nih.gov/pmc/articles/pmc2944261

Dayton, Tian. "Are You Self Medicating Your Emotional Stress with Food?" *Huffington Post Healthy Living*, November 17, 2011.

De Bloom, Jessica, et al. "Vacation (After-) Effects on Employee Health and Well-Being and the Role of Vacation Activities, Experiences and Sleep." *Journal of Happiness*, May 2012. DOI: 10.1007/S10902-012-9345-3

De Vries, Sjerp, Robert A. Verheij, and Peter P. Groenewegen. "Nature and Health: The Relation Between Health and Green Space in People's Living Environment." Paper presented at the Conference Cultural Events and Leisure Systems, Amsterdam, The Netherlands, April 2001.

Dell, Michael S. "Commencement Address 2003." 2003. www.utexas.edu/commence ment/2003/spring/speech.html

Department for Environment, Food & Rural Affairs. "The Natural Choice: Securing the Value of Nature. Presented to Parliament by the Secretary of State for Environment, Food and Rural Affairs, by Command of Her Majesty." United Kingdom, 2011.

Desbordes, Gaëlle. "Effects of Mindful-Attention and Compassion Meditation Training on Amygdala Response to Emotional Stimuli in an Ordinary, Non-Meditative State." *Frontiers in Human Neuroscience*, 2012; 6: 292. DOI: 10.3380/fnhum.2012.00292

Devries, Linda K. *Insomnia: Don't Lose Sleep Over It . . . Find the Help You Need.* Chicago: Harold Shaw Publishers, 2000.

Dietary Guidelines Advisory Committee. "Scientific Report of 2015." Part A, Executive Summary. https://health.gov/dietaryguidelines/2015-scientific-report/pdfs/02-executive-summary.pdf

Doheny, Kathleen. "It's Never Too Early to Teach Kids the Activity Habit." *Healthday*, November 25, 2004.

Drake, C. J. "Caffeine Effects on Sleep Taken 0, 3, or 6 Hours Before Going to Bed." *Journal of Clinical Sleep Medicine*, November 15, 2013; 9(11): 1195-200.

Drake, Victoria. "Inflammation." Linus Pauling Institute. Micronutrient Information Center. Oregon State University, August 2010. http://lpi.oregonstate.edu/mic/micronutrients-health/inflammation

Ekelund, Ulf, et al. "Physical Activity and All-Cause Mortality Across Levels of Overall and Abdominal Adiposity in European Men and Women: The European Prospective Investigation into Cancer and Nutrition Study (EPIC)." *American Journal of Clinical Exercise*, 2015; 1. DOI: 10.3945/Ajcn.114.100065

Emerman, Ed. "Companies Are Spending More on Corporate Wellness Programs but Employees Are Leaving Millions on the Table." *Business Group Health*, March 26, 2015.

Eng, Monica. "Light from Electronic Screens at Night Linked to Sleep Loss." *Chicago Tribune,* July 8, 2012.

Erickson, Kirk I. "Exercise Training Increases Size of Hippocampus and Improves Memory." *Proceedings of the National Academy of Sciences,* 2011; 108(7): 3017–22. DOI: 10.1073/Pnas.1015950108

Evans, Lisa. "Want More Sleep (and Better Productivity)? Work from Home." *Entrepreneur Magazine,* February 17, 2015.

Expedia. "2015 Vacation Deprivation Study: Europe Leads World in Paid Vacation Time While Americans and Asians Lag." November 26, 2015.

Fahkry, Tony. *The Power to Navigate Your Life.* Victoria, Australia: Heart Space Publications, 2014.

Farshchi, Hamid R. "Deleterious Effects of Omitting Breakfast on Insulin Sensitivity and Fasting Lipid Profiles in Healthy Lean Women." American Society for Clinical Nutrition. http://ajcn.nutrition.org/content/81/2/388. abstract.

Faux, Zeke. "Sweaty Wall Streeters Skip Booze for Spinclass Meetings." *Bloomberg Business,* July 18, 2013.

Federal Deposit Insurance Corporation. "Vacation Policies FIL-52-95." August 3, 1995.

Fielding, Thomas (John Wade). *Select Proverbs of All Nations.* 1824.

Fisher, R., et al. "Stand Up for Health—Avoiding Sedentary Behaviour Might Lengthen Your Telomeres: Secondary Outcomes from a Physical Activity RCT in Older People." *British Journal of Sports Medicine,* 2014; 48(19): 1407–9.

Fitzpatrick, A. L., et al. "Midlife and Late-Life Obesity and the Risk of Dementia: Cardiovascular Health Study." *Archives of Neurology,* 2009; 66: 336–42.

Fodor, Kate. "25 Surprising Ways Stress Affects Your Health." *Health.* http://www.health.com/health/gallery/0,,20642595,00.html

Fredrickson, Barbara L., et al. "Open Hearts Build Lives: Positive Emotions, Induced Through Loving-Kindness Meditation, Build Consequential Personal Resources." *The Journal of Personality and Social Psychology,* November 2008; 95(5): 1045–62. DOI: 10.1037/A0013262

Freeman, M. P. "Omega-3 Fatty Acids in Major Depressive Disorder." *Journal of Clinical Psychiatry,* 2009; 70(Suppl 5): 7 11. DOI: 10.4088/Jcp.8157sul C.02

Fresh, directed by Ana Sofia Joanes, Ripple Effect Films, 2009.

Fryer, Bronwyn. "Are You Working Too Hard?" *Harvard Business Review,* November 2005.

Fryer, Bronwyn. "Sleep Deficit: The Performance Killer." *Harvard Business Review,* October 2006.

Fuller, Patrick M., Jun Lu, and Clifford B. Saper. "Differential Rescue of Light- and Food-Entrainable Circadian Rhythms." *Science,* May 23, 2008; 320(5879): 1074–77. DOI: 10.1126/Science.1153277

Fung, T. T., V. Malik, K. M. Rexrode, J. E. Manson, W. C. Willett, and F. B. Hu. "Sweetened Beverage Consumption and Risk of Coronary Heart Disease in Women." *The American Journal of Clinical Nutrition,* 2009; 89: 1037–42.

Galinsky, Adam D. "Fashion with a Foreign Flair: Professional Experiences Abroad Facilitate the Creative Innovations of Organizations." *Academy of Management Journal*, May 2014; 58(1): 195–220.

Gallup-Healthways. "Well-being Index," 2008.

Gammon, Katharine. "Why Loneliness Can Be Deadly." *Livescience*, March 2012. www.livescience.com/18800-loneliness-health-problems.html

Gearhardt, M. S., and N. Ashley. "An Examination of the Food Addiction Construct in Obese Patients with Binge Eating Disorder." *International Journal of Eating Disorders*, July 2012; 45(5): 657–63.

Gelles, David. "The Mind Business." *Financial Times*, August 24, 2012.

Gibson, G. R., H. M. Probert, J. Van Loo, R. A. Rastall, and M. B. Roberfroid. "Dietary Modulation of the Human Colonic Microbiota: Updating the Concept of Prebiotics." *Nutrition Research Reviews*, 2004; 17(2): 259–75.

Glassdoor Employment Confidence Survey. "Average U.S. Employee Only Takes Half of Earned Vacation Time." April 3, 2014.

Global Business Travel Association. "U.S. Business Travel Marketplace to Remain Stable and Steady Despite Sea of Global Volatility." January 12, 2016.

Global Wellness Institute. "Global Spa & Wellness Economy Monitor." January 2015.

Global Wellness Institute. "Statistics & Facts." http://www.globalwellnessinstitute.org/statistics-and-facts/

Godbey, Geoffrey. "Outdoor Recreation, Health, and Wellness: Understanding and Enhancing the Relationship." *Resources for the Future*, May 2009.

Gold, M. S., K. Frost-Pineda, and W. S. Jacobs. "Overeating, Binge Eating, and Eating Disorders as Addictions." *Psychiatric Annals*, February 2003; 33(2): 117–22.

Goldman Sachs. "Millennial Impact Study." 2014. http://www.goldmansachs.com/our-thinking/pages/millennials/

Goldman Sachs. "Millennials: Coming of Age." http://www.goldmansachs.com/our-thinking/pages/millennials/

Gottlieb, D. J., et al. "Novel Loci Associated with Usual Sleep Duration: The CHARGE Consortium Genome-Wide Association Study." *Molecular Psychiatry*, October 2015; 20(10): 1232–39. DOI: 10.1038/Mp.2014.133. Epub December 2, 2014

Gow, Alan J. "Neuroprotective Lifestyles and the Aging Brain." *Neurology*, October 23, 2012; 79(17): 1802–8. DOI: http://dx.doi.org/10.1212/WNL.0b013e3182703fd2

Goyal, Madhav. "Mediation Programs of Psychological Stress and Well-Being." *JAMA Internal Medicine*, 2014; 174(3): 357–68.

Gram, Martin, et al. "Two Weeks of One-leg Immobilization Decreases Skeletal Muscle Respiratory Capacity Equally in Young and Elderly Men." *Experimental Gerontology*, 2014; 58(10): 269–78.

Graves, Ginny. "10 Strategies for a More Restful Night's Sleep." *Allure Magazine*, 2008; 9(11):1195–200.

Groesz, Lisa, et al. "What Is Eating You? Stress and the Drive to Eat." *Appetite*, April 2012; 58(2): 717–21.

Gump, B., and K. Matthews. "Are Vacations Good for Your Health? The 9-Year Mortality Experience after the Multiple Risk Factor Intervention Trial." *Psychosomatic Medicine*, 2000; 62(5): 608–12.

Gupta, Sanjay. "Why You Should Treat Loneliness as a Chronic Illness." *Everyday Health*, August 4, 2015.

Haiken, Melanie. "The New Theory on Weight Loss: Your Bad Diet Has Damaged Your Brain." *Forbes*, August 21, 2013.

Hair, Marilyn and Jon Sharpe. "Fast Facts About the Human Microbiome," The Center for Ecogenetics and Environmental Health. University of Washington, January 2014.

Hallowell, Edward. "Overloaded Circuits: Why Smart People Underperform." *Harvard Business Review*, January 2005.

Hamilton, Elizabeth. "Feel Groggy in the Mornings? Here's How to Wake Up Refreshed." *Dallas Morning News*, February 16, 2015.

Hanh, Thich Nhat. *Cultivating the Mind of Love*. Berkeley, CA: Parallax Press, 1996.

Hansen, Anita L. "Fish Consumption, Sleep, Daily Functioning, and Heart Rate Variability," American Academy of Sleep Medicine. University of Bergen, Norway, 2014.

Harris, Shelby Freedman. "6 Ways Sleep Makes Your Life Better." *The Huffington Post Healthy Living*, September 14, 2014. http://www.huffingtonpost.com/2014/09/14/benefits-of-sleep_n_5799214.html

Hartzler, Beth. "Fatigue on the Flight Deck: The Consequences of Sleep Loss and the Benefits of Napping." *Accident Analysis and Prevention*, January 2014; 62: 309–18. DOI: 10.1016/J.Aap.2013.10.010. Epub October 19, 2013.

Harvard Medical School. "Insomnia: Restoring Restful Sleep. The Family Health Guide." *Harvard Medical Publications*, March 2009.

Harvard Medical School. "Newsletter." July 2010. http://www.health.harvard.edu/news-letters/harvard_health_letter/2010/july

Harvard Medical School. "Sleep and Disease Risk." December 2007. http://healthysleep.med.harvard.edu/healthy/matters/consequences/sleep-and-disease-risk

Harvard School of Public Health. "Coffee by the Numbers." 2010. http://www.hsph.harvard.edu/news/multimedia-article/facts/

Healthday News. "The Weird Reason People Snack More While Watching Action Movies." September 2, 2014. http://news.health.com/2014/09/02/Action-Packed-Tv-A-Threat-To-Your-Waistline/

Hemp, Paul. "Presenteeism: At Work—But Out of It." *Harvard Business Review*, October 2004.

Herxheimer, A. "Melatonin for the Prevention and Treatment of Jet Lag." *Cochrane Database Systematic Review*, 2002; (2): CD001520. http://www.ncbi.nlm.nih.gov/pubmed/12076414

Higgins, Janine A. "Resistant Starch and Exercise Independently Attenuate Weight Regain on a High Fat Diet in a Rat Model of Obesity." *Nutrition & Metabolism*, July 7, 2011; 8. DOI:10.1186/1743-7075-8-49

Hildebrandt, M. A., et al. "High Fat Diet Determines the Composition of the Murine Gut Microbiome Independently of Obesity." *Gastroenterology*, 2009; 137(5): 1716–24.

Hines, Ree. "Oprah Unveils Her Weight-loss Transformation, Talks 'Best Body' in O." *Today*, March 11, 2016.

His Holiness the Dalai Lama. *The Path to Tranquility: Daily Meditations*. New York: Penguin Books, 1998.

Hochman, David. "Mindfulness: Getting Its Share of Attention." *The New York Times*, November 1, 2013.

Hoffman, Benson M., et al. "Exercise and Pharmacotherapy in Patients with Major Depression: One-year Follow-up of the Smile Study." *Psychosomatic Medicine*, February–March 2011; 73(2): 127–33. DOI: 10.1097/Psy.0b013e31820433a5. Epub December 10, 2010.

Hoge, Elizabeth. "Mindfulness and Self-Compassion in Generalize Anxiety Disorder." *Evidence-based Complementary and Alternative Medicine*, 2013; 34–40. DOI: 10.1155/2013/576258

Holt-Lunstad, J., T. B. Smith, and J. B. Layton. "Social Relationships and Mortality Risk: A Meta-Analytic Review." *PLoS Medicine*, 2010; 7(7): E1000316. DOI:10.1371/Journal.Pmed.1000316

Hopkins, M. E. "Differential Effects of Acute and Regular Physical Exercise on Cognition and Affect." *Neuroscience*, July 26, 2012; 215: 59–68. DOI: 10.1016/j.neuroscience.2012.04.056. Epub April 30, 2012.

Horovitz, Bruce. "Younger Folks Want Healthier Food—And Will Pay for It." *USA Today*, January 19, 2015.

Huffington, Arianna. "Mindfulness, Meditation, Wellness and Their Connection to Corporate America's Bottom Line." *The Huffington Post*, March 18, 2013.

Huffington, Arianna. "My Q and A with Michael Breus, aka the Sleep Doctor." *The Huffington Post*, September 8, 2015. http://www.huffingtonpost.com/arianna-huffington/my-q-and-a-with-michael-breus-aka-the-sleep-doctor_b_8104520.html

Huth, C., et al. "Job Strain as a Risk Factor for the Onset of Type 2 Diabetes Mellitus: Findings from the MONICA/KORA Augsburg Cohort Study." *Psychosomatic Medicine*, September 2014; 76(7): 562–68. DOI: 10.1097/PSY.0000000000000084

Hyman, Mark. "10 Dramatic Shifts That Occur When You Detox." July 2015. http://drhyman.com/blog/2015/07/03/10-dramatic-shifts-that-occur-when-you-detox/

Hyman, Mark. "10 Strategies to Eat Healthy While You Travel." June 26, 2015. http://drhyman.com/blog/2015/06/25/10-strategies-to-eat-healthy-while-you-travel/

IARC. "Painting, Firefighting, and Shiftwork: IARC Monographs on the Evaluation of Carcinogenic Risks to Humans." Vol. 98. Lyon, France: International Agency for Research on Cancer, Working Group on the Evaluation of Carcinogenic Risks to Humans, 2007.

"IDC Forecasts Worldwide Shipments of Wearables to Surpass 200 Million in 2019, Driven by Strong Smartwatch Growth." *IDC Worldwide Quarterly*, December 17, 2015. https://www.idc.com/getdoc.jsp?containerId=prUS41100116

In Defense of Food, by Michael Pollan, directed by Michael Schwarz, 2015.

Inniss, A. M., B. L. Rice, and S. M. Smith. "Dietary Support of Extended-Duration Bed Rest Studies." *International Journal of Workplace Health Management*, 2006. https://ntrs.nasa.gov/archive/nasa/casi.ntrs.nasa.gov/20060018323.pdf

Ishige, K. "Flavonoids Protect Neuronal Cells from Oxidative Stress by Three Distinct Mechanisms." *Free Radical Biology and Medicine*, February 15, 2001; 30(4): 433–46.

Jacka, F. N., N. Cherbuin, K. J. Anstey, and P. Butterworth. "Dietary Patterns and Depressive Symptoms Over Time: Examining the Relationships with Socioeconomic Position, Health Behaviours and Cardiovascular Risk." *PLoS One*, 2014; 9(1): E87657. DOI:10.1371/Journal.Pone.008765

Jacobs, J. M. "Going Outdoors Daily Predicts Long-term Functional and Health Benefits among Ambulatory Older People." *Journal of Aging and Health*, April 2008; 20(3): 259–72. DOI: 10.1177/0898264308315427

Jacobs, T. L., et al. "Intensive Meditation Training, Immune Cell Telomerase Activity, and Psychological Mediators." *Psychoneuroendocrinology*, 2010; 36(5): 664–81. DOI: 10.1016/J.Psyneuen.2010.09.010

Jacobsen, Maryann Tomovich. "Juices: The Best and Worst for Your Health." *WebMD*, May 2014. http://www.webmd.com/diet/ss/slideshow-juice-wars

Jensen, Eric. *Learning with the Body in Mind*. Thousand Oaks, CA: Corwin Press, 2000.

Johnson, Carla. "Preventing Colds May Be as Easy as Vitamin Zzz Updated." Associated Press, January 2009.

Jones, Jeffrey M. "In U.S., 40% Get Less than Recommended Amount of Sleep." *Gallup*, December 19, 2013. http://www.gallup.com/poll/166553/less-recommended-amount-sleep.aspx

Juster, F. T., F. Stafford, and H. Ono. *Changing Times of American Youth: 1981–2003*. Institute for Social Research, Ann Arbor, MI: University of Michigan. http://www.ns.umich.edu/releases/2004/Nov04/teen_time_report.pdf

Kabat-Zinn, J., L. Lipworth, and R. Burney. "The Clinical Use of Mindfulness Meditation for the Self-Regulation of Chronic Pain." *Journal of Behavioral Medicine*, June 1985; 8(2): 163–90.

Kahan, V. "Can Poor Sleep Affect Skin Integrity?" *Medical Hypotheses*, December 2010; 75(6): 535–37. DOI: 10.1016/J.Mehy.2010.07.018. Epub August 1, 2010. http://www.ncbi.nlm.nih.gov/pubmed/20678867

Kaiser Family Foundation. "2014 Employer Health Benefits Survey." Kaiser/HRET, 2004–2014, September 2014.

Kaplan, Rachel, and Stephen Kaplan. *The Experience of Nature: A Psychological Perspective*. Cambridge: Cambridge University Press, 1989.

Karl, T., et al. "Y1 Receptors Regulate Aggressive Behavior by Modulating Serotonin Pathways." *Proceedings of the National Academy of Sciences of the United States of America*, August 24, 2004; 101(34): 12742–47.

Karmin, Craig. "Equinox Fitness Clubs Expand to Hotels." *The Wall Street Journal*, April 2015.

Kasem, Casey. "Casey Kasem's Final American Top 20 Broadcast." July 2009. https://www.youtube.com/watch?v=lCxq6vjAvWs

Kessler, R. C., et al. "Insomnia and the Performance of U.S. Workers: Results from the America Insomnia Survey." *Sleep*, September 1, 2011; 34(9): 1161–71. DOI: 10.5665/SLEEP.1230

Khazan, Olga. "Why It Was Easier to Be Skinny in the 1980s." *The Atlantic*, September 30, 2015.

Kim, Sangmi. "Eating Patterns and Nutritional Characteristics Associated with Sleep Duration." *Public Health Nutrition*, May 2011; 14(5): 889–95. Published online October 29, 2010. DOI: 10.1017/S136898001000296X, PMCID: PMC3179429 NIHMSID: NIHMS322771. https://www.ncbi.nlm.nih.gov/pmc/articles/pmc3179429/

Kim, W., S. K. Lim, E. J. Chung, and J. M. Woo. "The Effect of Cognitive Behavior Therapy Based Psychotherapy Applied in a Forest Environment on Psychological Changes and Remission of Major Depression." *Psychiatry Investigation*, 2009; 6: 245–54.

Klepeis, Neil E. "The National Human Activity Pattern Survey (NHAPS): A Resource for Assessing Exposure to Environmental Pollutants." *Journal of Exposure Analysis and Environmental Epidemiology*, 2001; 11: 231–52. DOI: 10.1038/Sj.Jea.7500165

Knutson, K. L., A. M. Ryden, V. A. Mander, and E. Van Cauter. "Role of Sleep Duration and Quality in the Risk and Severity of Type 2 Diabetes Mellitus." *Archives of Internal Medicine*, 2006; 166: 1768–64.

Koenig, H. G. "Religious Attitudes and Practices of Hospitalized Medically Ill Older Adults." *International Journal of Geriatric Psychiatry*, April 1998; 13(4): 213–24.

Kohl, Harold W. "The Pandemic of Physical Inactivity: Global Action for Public Health." *The Lancet*, July 18, 2012; 380(9838): 294–305. DOI: http://dx.doi.org/10.1016/S0140-6736(12)60898-8

Konczak, Izabela. "Anthocyanins—More Than Nature's Colours." *Journal of Biomedicine and Biotechnology*, December 1, 2004; 5: 239–40. DOI: 10-1155-S111 0724304407013, Pmcid Pmc1082903

Konnikova, Maria. "Why Can't We Fall Asleep?" *New Yorker*, July 7, 2015.

Korn, Melissa. "Smartphones Make You Tired and Unproductive, Study Says." *Wall Street Journal*, February 6, 2014.

Kotzampassi, K., and E. J. Giamarellos-Bourboulis. "Probiotics for Infectious Diseases: More Drugs, Less Dietary Supplementation." *International Journal of Antimicrobial Agents*, 2012; 40: 288–96.

Kross, E., et al. "Facebook Use Predicts Declines in Subjective Well-being in Young Adults." *PLoS One*, 2013; 8(8): E69841. DOI: 10.1371/Journal.Pone.0069841

Kulkarni, A. A. "Associations Between Diet Quality and Mental Health in Socially Disadvantaged New Zealand Adolescents." *European Journal of Clinical Nutrition*, January 2015; 69(1): 7983. DOI: 10.1038/Ejcn.2014.130. Epub July 16, 2014

Kuo, F., and A. Taylor. "A Potential Natural Treatment for Attention-Deficit/Hyperactivity Disorder: Evidence from a National Study." *American Journal of Public Health*, 2004; 94(9): 1580–86.

Lee, I-Min. "Physical Activity and Weight Gain Prevention." *JAMA*, 2010; 303(12): 1173–79. DOI: 10.1001/Jama.2010.312

Lenoir, M., F. Serre, L. Cantin, and S. H. Ahmed. "Intense Sweetness Surpasses Cocaine Reward." *PLoS One*, 2007; 2(8): E698. DOI: 10.1371/Journal.Pone.0000698

Lerman, Katrina. "Healthcare Without Borders: How Millennials Are Reshaping Health and Wellness." *Communispace*, August 1, 2014. https://healthcaresocialmedia.files. wordpress.com/2014/11/how-millennials-are-reshaping-digital-health.png

Lewine, Howard. "Too Little Sleep, and Too Much, Affect Memory." *Harvard Health Blog*, May 2014. http://www.health.harvard.edu/blog/little-sleep-much-affect-memory-201405027136

Lewis, Steven and Charles H. Hennekens. "Regular Physical Activity: Forgotten Benefits." *The American Journal of Medicine*, February 2016; 129(2). DOI: 10.1016/J. Amjmed.2015.07.016

Li, Qing. "Acute Effects of Walking in Forest Environments on Cardiovascular and Metabolic Parameters." *European Journal of Applied Physiology*, 2011; 111: 2845–53. DOI: 10.1007/S00421-011-1918-Z

Li, Qing. "Visiting a Forest, but Not a City, Increases Human Natural Killer Activity and Expression of Anticancer Proteins." *International Journal of Immunopathology and Pharmacology*, January–March 2008; 21(1): 117–27.

Lin, F. "Effect of Different Sitting Postures on Lung Capacity, Expiratory Flow, and Lumbar Lordosis." *The Archives of Physical Medicine and Rehabilitation*, April 2006; 87(4): 504–9.

Lipman, Frank. "How Do I Stay Calm with All the Stress in My Life?" Blog, January 4, 2011. www.drfranklipman.com

Lisle, Douglas J. "Break Your Food Addictions." *WebMD*. http://www.webmd.com/food-recipes/features/breaking-food-adictions#1

Liu, Bor-Shong, and Chia-Chen Wu. "Survey of Health Problems for Long-Haul Flight Travelers." Department of Industrial Engineering and Management, St. John's University. Project No. Nsc 98-2221-E-129-003.

Lockley, Steven W., et al. "Effect of Reducing Interns' Weekly Work Hours on Sleep and Attentional Failures." *The New England Journal of Medicine*, October 28, 2004; 351: 1829–37. DOI: 10.1056/NEJMoa041404

Louv, Richard. *Last Child in the Woods: Saving Our Children from Nature-Deficit Disorder*. New York: Workman Publishing Company, 2005.

Lovato, Nicole. "Evaluation of a Brief Treatment Program of Cognitive Behavior Therapy for Insomnia in Older Adults." *Sleep*, 2014; 37(1): 117–26. http://dx.doi.org/10.5665/sleep.3320

Luders, Eileen, Nicolas Cherbuin, and Florian Kurth. "Forever Young(er): Potential Age-Defying Effects of Long-term Meditation on Gray Matter Atrophy." *Frontiers in Psychology*, 2014; 5: 1551. Published online January 21, 2015. DOI: 10.3389/fpsyg.2014.01551. http://journal.frontiersin.org/article/10.3389/fpsyg.2014.01551/full

Luppino, F. S., et al. "Overweight, Obesity, and Depression: A Systematic Review and Meta-analysis of Longitudinal Studies." *Archives of General Psychiatry*, 2010; 67: 220–29.

Macht, M. "Immediate Effects of Chocolate on Experimentally Induced Mood States." *Appetite*, November 2007; 49(3): 667–74. Epub May 23, 2007.

Mackenzie, Corey S., Patricia A. Poulin, and Rhonda Seidman-Carlson. "A Brief Mindfulness-Based Stress Reduction Intervention for Nurses and Nurse Aides." *Applied Nursing Research*, 2006; 19: 105–9.

Maclean, P. S. "Regular Exercise Attenuates the Metabolic Drive to Regain Weight After Longterm Weight Loss." *American Journal of Physiology—Regulatory, Integrative and Comparative Physiology*, September 2009; 297(3): R793802. DOI: 10.1152/Ajpregu.00192.2009. Epub July 8, 2009.

Mark, Gloria J., and Stephen Voida. "A Pace Not Dictated by Electrons: An Empirical Study of Work Without Email." Department of Informatics, University of California, Irvine. https://www.ics.uci.edu/gmark/home_page/research_files/chi%202012.pdf

Mattke, Soeren, et al. "Workplace Wellness Program Study." *RAND Health*, 2013.

Mauskop, Alexander and Jasmine Varughese. "Why All Migraine Patients Should Be Treated with Magnesium." *Journal of Neural Transmission*, May 2012; 119(5): 575–79.

Mayerowitz, Scott. "How to Beat Jet Lag." *Travel and Leisure Magazine*, August 2015. www.travelandleisure.com/articles/how-to-beat-jet-lag

Mayo Clinic. "HDL Cholesterol: How to Boost Your 'Good' Cholesterol." November 2012. http://www.mayoclinic.org/diseases-conditions/high-blood-cholesterol/in-depth/hdl-cholesterol/art-20046388?pg=2

Mayo Clinic Staff. "Exercise: 7 Benefits of Regular Physical Activity." February 2014. http://www.mayoclinic.org/healthy-lifestyle/fitness/in-depth/exercise/art-20048389

McClelland, David C. *Human Motivation*. Cambridge: Cambridge University Press, 1987.

McGreevey, Sue. "Eight Weeks to a Better Brain." *Harvard Gazette*, January 21, 2011.

McGregor, Jenna. "The Average Worker Loses 11 Days of Productivity Each Year Due to Insomnia, and Companies are Taking Notice." *Washington Post*, July 30, 2015.

McMullen, Tom. "Enabling, Engaging, & Rewarding Employees." *Hay Group*, Mexico City, April 6, 2011.

McPherson, Miller, et al. "Social Isolation in America: Changes in Core Discussion Networks Over Two Decades." *American Sociological Review*, June 2006; 71: 353–75.

Medical Dictionary. S.v. "enriched food." Retrieved April 1, 2016, from http://medical-dictionary.thefreedictionary.com/enriched+food

Mednick, Sara C. "Comparing the Benefits of Caffeine, Naps and Placebo on Verbal, Motor and Perceptual Memory." *Behavioural Brain Research*, November 3, 2008; 193(1): 79–86.

Mejia, Robin. "Green Exercise May Be Good for Your Head." *Environmental Science and Technology*, April 21, 2010; 44. http://pubs.acs.org/doi/full/10.1021/Es101129n

Meltzer, Marisa. "Why Fitness Classes Are Making You Go Broke." *Racked.Com*, June 10, 2015. http://www.racked.com/2015/6/10/8748149/fitness-class-costs

Men in Black, directed by Barry Sonnenfeld, Columbia Pictures, 1997.

Merchant, Nilofer. "Got a Meeting? Take a Walk." *TED*, 2013. www.ted.com/talks/nilofer_merchant_got_a_meeting_take_a_walk?language=en

Mercola, Joseph. "This Is What Happens to Your Body When You Exercise." *Peak Fitness*, September 20, 2013.

Merriam-Webster. "Intuition." http://www.merriam-webster.com/dictionary/intuition

Michigan State University. "Virtual Workout Partners Spur Better Results, Study Finds." *ScienceDaily*. www.sciencedaily.com/releases/2011/05/110518161707.htm

"Millennial Consumer Study 2015." *Elite Daily*, January 19, 2015. http://elitedaily.com/news/business/elite-daily-millennial-consumer-survey-2015/

Milligan, Susan. "The Limits of Unlimited Vacation." *Society for Human Resources Management*, March 2015; 60(2).

Milne, A. A. *When We Were Very Young*. New York: Puffin Books, 1924. Reissue edition August 1, 1992.

Mintel. "Fitness Fuels US Consumer Desire for Wearable Tech with Sales Increasing 186% in 2015." January 2016. www.idc.com/getdoc.jsp?containerid=prus40846515

Mintel. "Voyage of Discovery as Education Becomes Latest Travel Trend." September 11, 2009. http://www.mintel.com/press-centre/travel/voyage-of-discovery-as-education-becomes-latest-travel-trend

More, T., and B. Payne. "Affective Responses to Natural Areas Near Cities." *Journal of Leisure Research*, 1978; 10(1): 7–12.

Morning Edition, NPR. "Gut Bacteria Might Guide the Workings of Our Minds." November 18, 2013. http://www.npr.org/sections/health-shots/2013/11/18/244526773/gut-bacteria-might-guide-the-workings-of-our-minds

Moss, Michael. *Salt Sugar Fat: How the Food Giants Hooked Us*. New York: Random House, 2013.

Moss, Michael. "The Extraordinary Science of Addictive Junk Food." *The New York Times Magazine*, February 2013.

Motluk, Alison. "Meditation Builds Up the Brain." *New Scientist*, November 2005.

Murphy, Margi. "Why Intel's Latest Purchase and Fitbit's £3.8bn Valuation Prove Wearables Aren't a Fad." *Techworld*, June 19, 2015. http://www.techworld.com/wearables/wearables-are-not-fad-why-intels-latest-purchase-fitbits-ipo-are-proof-3616271/

Myers, Jonathan. "Exercise and Cardiovascular Health." *American Heart Association*, 2003. DOI: 10.1161/01.CIR.0000048890.59383.8D

National Center for Complementary and Integrative Health. "Use of Complementary Health Approaches in the U.S." February 2015. https://nccih.nih.gov/research/statistics/NHIS/2012/mind-body/yoga

National Heart, Lung, and Blood Institute. "Why Is Sleep Important?" February 2012. http://www.nhlbi.nih.gov/health/health-topics/topics/sdd/why

National Institutes of Mental Health. "Any Anxiety Disorder Among Adults." http://www.nimh.nih.gov/health/statistics/prevalence/file_148008.pdf

National Sleep Foundation. "Sleep-Wake Cycle: Its Physiology and Impact on Health." 2006. https://sleepfoundation.org/sites/default/files/SleepWakeCycle.pdf

Nawijn, Jeroen, et al. "Vacationers Happier, but Most Not Happier After a Holiday." *Applied Research Quality Life*, February 2010; 5: 35–47. DOI: 10.1007/S11482-009-9091-9

Neiger, Chris. "9 Facts You Didn't Know about Wearable Technology." *The Motley Fool*, February 15, 2016. http://www.fool.com/investing/general/2016/02/15/9-facts-you-didnt-know-about-wearable-technology.aspx

Nesse, Randolph and George Williams. *Why We Get Sick: The New Science of Darwinian Medicine.* New York: Vintage, 1996.

New York Blue Light Symposium. "Welcome Message." June 2015. http://blue-light.biz/2isbls/img/Panf-2isbls.pdf

Nielsen, Global Health & Wellness Report. "We Are What We Eat: Healthy Eating Trends Around the World." January 2015. https://www.nielsen.com/content/dam/nielsenglobal/eu/nielseninsights/pdfs/nielsen%20global%20health%20and%20wellness%20report%20-%20january%202015.pdf

Nielsen, Tore. "Dreams of the Rarebit Fiend: Food and Diet as Instigators of Bizarre and Disturbing Dreams." *Frontiers in Psychology*, February 17, 2015. http://dx.doi.org/10.3389/fpsyg.2015.00047

Northup, Temple. "Understanding the Relationship between Television Use and Unhealthy Eating: The Mediating Role of Fatalistic Views of Eating Well and Nutritional Knowledge." *The International Journal of Communication and Health*, 2014; 3: 10.

Nowson Ca, et al. "Vitamin D and Health in Adults in Australia and New Zealand: A Position Statement." *Medical Journal of Australia*, 2012; 196(11): 686–87.

O'Brien, James. "Understanding the Digital Habits of Millennial Business Travelers." *Skift*, November 2014.

O'Brien, Jennifer. "UCSF Study on Multitasking Reveals Switching Glitch in Aging Brain." 2011. https://www.ucsf.edu/news/2011/04/9676/ucsf-study-multitasking-reveals-switching-glitch-aging-brain

Oppezzo, Marily. "Give Your Ideas Some Legs: The Positive Effect of Walking on Creative Thinking." *Stanford University Journal of Experimental Psychology Learning Memory and Cognition*, July 2014; 40(4): 1142–52. DOI: 10.1037/A0036577. Epub April 21, 2014.

Owens, Judith A., et al. "Impact of Delaying School Start Time on Adolescent Sleep, Mood, and Behavior." *Archives of Pediatrics Adolescent Medicine*, July 2010; 164(7): 608–14. DOI: 10.1001/Archpediatrics.2010.96

Parajuli, Ashutosh. "Bone's Responses to Mechanical Loading are Impaired in Type 1 Diabetes." *Bone*. Published online: July 13, 2015. DOI: http://Dx.Doi.Org/10.1016/J.Bone.2015.07.012

Park, Bum-Jin. "Physiological Effects of Shinrin-Yoku (Taking in the Atmosphere of the Forest)—Using Salivary Cortisol and Cerebral Activity as Indicators." *Journal of Physiology Anthropology*, 2006; 26(2): 123–28. DOI: 10.2114/Jpa2.26.123

Park, Bum-Jin. "Using Salivary Cortisol and Cerebral Activity as Indicators." *Journal of Physiological Anthropology*, 2006; 26(2): 123–28.

Parker, Ian. "The Big Sleep." *New Yorker*, December 9, 2013. http://www.newyorker.com/magazine/2013/12/09/the-big-sleep-2

Parry, Thomas. "Total Lost-Time Management: The Link between Absence and Presenteeism." *Integrated Benefits Institute*, June 2008.

Parvez, S., et al. "Probiotics and Their Fermented Food Products Are Beneficial for Health." *Journal of Applied Microbiology*, April 2006. DOI: 10.1111/J.1365-2672.2006.02963.X

Passos, G. S. "Effects of Moderate Aerobic Exercise Training on Chronic Primary Insomnia." *Sleep Medicine*, December 2011; 12(10): 101827. DOI: 10.1016/J. Sleep.2011.02.007

Peltier, Dan. "Business Travelers Unsure If 'Bleisure' Travel Is Allowed, but Doing It Anyway." *Skift*, October 22, 2014. https://skift.com/2014/10/22/business-travelers-unsure-if-bleisure-travel-is-allowed-but-doing-it-anyway/

Pergams, O. R. W., and P. A. Zaradic. "Evidence for a Fundamental and Pervasive Shift Away from Nature Based Recreation." *Proceedings of the National Academy of Sciences*, 2007; 105: 2295–300. DOI: 10.1073/Pnas.0709893105

Perlow, Leslie A. "Overcome Your Work Addiction." *Harvard Business Review*, May 2, 2012. https://hbr.org/2012/05/overcome-your-work-addiction.html

Pinsker, Joe. "Corporations' Newest Productivity Hack: Meditation." *The Atlantic*, March 10, 2015. http://www.theatlantic.com/business/archive/2015/03/corporations-newest-productivity-hack-meditation/387286/

Planells, E. "Effect of Magnesium Deficiency on Vitamin B2 and B6 Status in the Rat." *Journal of the American College of Nutrition*, August 1997; 16(4): 352–56.

Population Reference Bureau. "World Population Highlights 2007:Urbanization." September 2007. http://www.prb.org/publications/datasheets/2007/2007worldpopulationdatasheet.aspx

Potera, Carol. "Diet and Nutrition: The Artificial Food Dye Blues." *Environmental Health Perspectives*, October 2010; 118(10): A428. DOI: 10.1289/Ehp.118-A428

Poulain, Michel and Giovanni Mario Pes. "Identification of a Geographic Area Characterized by Extreme Longevity in the Sardinia Island: The Akea Study." *Experimental Gerontology*, September 2004; 39(9): 1423–29.

Pretty, J. "The Mental and Physical Health Outcomes of Green Exercise." *International Journal of Environmental Health Research*, October 2005; 15(5): 319–37.

Proal, A. D., P. J. Albert, and T. G. Marshall. "The Human Microbiome and Autoimmunity." *Current Opinion in Rheumatology*, March 2013; 25(2): 234–40. DOI: 10.1097/BOR.0b013e32835cedbf

Project: Time Off. "The Hidden Costs of Unused Leave." Oxford Economics Study, 2015.

Project: Time Off. "The Role of Business Travel in the U.S. Economy." 2013.

Project: Time Off. "The Work Martyr's Children: How Kids Are Harmed by America's Lost Week." September 2015. http://www.projecttimeoff.com/sites/default/files/PTO_WMC_Report.pdf

Public Health England. "Ecotherapy: The Green Agenda for Mental Health." (Exec. Summ.) *Mind*, UK. https://www.mind.org.uk/media/273470/ecotherapy.pdf

Puhan, Milo A. "Didgeridoo Playing as Alternative Treatment for Obstructive Sleep Apnea Syndrome: Randomized Controlled Trial." *British Medical Journal*, February 2006.

Plutchik, Michael, and Henry Kellerman, eds. *Biological Foundations of Emotion*. Cambridge, MA: Academic Press, 1986.

Queensland University of Technology. "Treating Sugar Addiction Like Drug Abuse." *Science Daily*, April 7, 2016. www.sciencedaily.com/releases/2016/04/160407111828.htm

Rabin, Roni Caryn. "Placing a Cap on Americans' Consumption of Added Sugar." *New York Times*, November 9, 2015.

Ramsey, Lydia. "The USDA Just Released a Massive New Report on What's Actually Healthy." *Business Insider*, January 7, 2016. http://www.businessinsider.com/usda-2015-guidelines-2016-12

Rangel-Huerta, O. D., C. M. Aguilera, M. D. Mesa, and A. Gil. "Omega-3 Long Chain Polyunsaturated Fatty Acids Supplementation on Inflammatory Biomakers: A Systematic Review of Randomized Clinical Trials." *British Journal of Nutrition*, 2012; 107: S159 70.

Rapoza, Kenneth. "Business Travel Market to Surpass $1 Trillion This Year." *Forbes*, August 6, 2013.

Ray, Rebecca, Milla Sanes, and John Schmitt. "No-Vacation Nation Revisited." Center for Economic and Policy Research, May 2013. http://cepr.net/publications/reports/no-vacation-nation-2013

Reaney, Patricia. "Global Spa, Wellness Industry Estimated at $3.4 Trillion." *Reuters*, September 30, 2014.

Rechtschaffen, Allan and Bernard Bergmann. "Sleep Deprivation in the Rat: An Update of the 1989 Paper." *Sleep*, 2002; 25(1): 18–24.

Reynolds, Gretchen. "Weighing the Evidence on Exercise." *New York Times Magazine*, April 16, 2010.

Richards, Catherine. "Business Travel and Self-Rated Health, Obesity, and Cardiovascular Disease Risk Factors." *Journal of Occupational & Environmental Medicine*, April 2011; 53(4): 358–63. DOI: 10.1097/Jom.0b013e3182143e77

Richter, Jean Paul, trans. "The Notebooks of Leonardo Da Vinci." 1888. www.gutenberg.org/cache/epub/5000/pg5000.html

Rideout, V. J., U. G. Foehr, and D. F. Roberts. "Generation M2: Media in the Lives of 8- to 18-year-olds." *The Henry J Kaiser Family Foundation Report*, January 20, 2010. http://www.kff.org/entmedia/8010.cfm

Robbins, Liz. "Great Workout, Forget the View." *New York Times*, February 18, 2009.

Rock, David and Jeffrey Schwartz. "The Neuroscience of Leadership." *Summer Strategy + Business*, May 30, 2006; 43. http://www.strategy-business.com/article/06207?gko=6da0a

Roenneberg, Till. "Is Light-at-Night a Health Risk Factor or a Health Risk Predictor?" *Chronobiology International: The Journal of Biological and Medical Rhythm Research*, 2009; 26(6). DOI: 10.3109/07420520903223984

Rohrmann, Sabine, et al. "Meat Consumption and Mortality—Results from the European Prospective Investigation into Cancer and Nutrition." *BMC Medicine*, 2013; 11(63). DOI: 10.1186/1741-7015-11-63

Rosekind, M. R. "Alertness Management: Strategic Naps in Operational Settings." *Journal of Sleep Research*, December 1995; 4(S2): 62–66. http://www.ncbi.nlm.nih.gov/pubmed/10607214

Rosenbloom, Stephanie. "A Battle Plan for Jet Lag." *The New York Times*, August 15, 2012.

Roth, T. "Prevalence, Associated Risks, and Treatment Patterns of Insomnia." *Journal of Clinical Psychiatry*, 2005; 66(Suppl 9): 10–13. Quiz 423.

Rowe, Albert H. *Elimination Diets and the Patient's Allergies: A Handbook of Allergy.* Philadelphia: Lea & Febiger, 1941.

Rubinstein, A., Y. Lurie, I. Groskop, and M. Weintrob. "Cholesterol-Lowering Effects of a 10 Mg Daily Dose of Lovastatin in Patients with Initial Total Cholesterol Levels 200 to 240 Mg/Dl (5.18 To 6.21 Mmol/Liter)." *American Journal of Cardiology*, November 1, 1991; 68(11): 1123–26. http://www.ncbi.nlm.nih.gov/pubmed/1951068

Ruppel, Glenn, Jim Avila, and Mark Greenblat. "Mice, Roaches Seen by FDA Inspecting Airline Food." *ABC News*, November 17, 2012.

Russell, Roly. "Humans and Nature: How Knowing and Experiencing Nature Affect Well Being." *Annual Review of Environment and Resources*, 2013; 38: 473. DOI: 10.1146/Annurev_Environ_012312_110838

Ryu, Ja Young. "Association Between Body Size Phenotype and Sleep Duration: Korean National Health and Nutrition Examination Survey V." December 1, 2014.

Sarris, Jerome. "Nutrients and Herbal Supplements for Mental Health." *Australian Prescriber*, June 2, 2014; 37: 90–93. http://dx.doi.org/10.18773/austprescr.2014.036

Savage, Stephanie. "Study Finds Warning Signs of Diabetes Can Show Up in Just a Few Days." *ABC Radio*, September 9, 2015.

Schaffer, Linden. "Simple Ways to Eat Clean for Overall Wellness." *The Huffington Post Healthy Living*, November 5, 2013.

Schaffer, Linden. "Well on the Road Interview." 2015/2016.

Schaffer, Linden. "Pravassa's Well on the Road Interview Series." www.pravassa.com.

Schneider, Robert. "Stress Reduction in the Secondary Prevention of Cardiovascular Disease." *American Heart Association Journals*, July 16, 2012. circoutcomes.ahajournals.org/content/5/6/750.abstract

Seidenberg, Casey. "Why Sugar and Caffeine Only Make Your Teen More Stressed During Cram Sessions." *Washington Post*, March 16, 2016.

Seneca, Lucius Annaeus. "Letter LXXXIV: On Gathering Ideas, Line 13—*Epistulae Morales ad Lucilium*" (Moral Letters to Lucilius).

Shah, Amy. "10 Reasons to Think Twice before Going to the Doctor." *mindbodygreen*, May 2, 2014. http://www.mindbodygreen.com/0-13606/10-reasons-to-think-twice-before-going-to-the-doctor-advice-from-an-md.html

Shariff, M., et al. "Neuronal Nicotinic Acetylcholine Receptor Modulators Reduce Sugar Intake." *PLoS ONE*, 2016; 11(3): E0150270. DOI: 10.1371/Journal.Pone.0150270

Sheiham, Aubrey, W. Philip, and T. James. "A Reappraisal of the Quantitative Relationship Between Sugar Intake and Dental Caries: The Need for New Criteria for

Developing Goals for Sugar Intake." *BMC Public Health.* DOI: 10.1186/1471-2458-14-863

Sheiham, Aubrey, W. Philip, and T. James. "A Reappraisal of the Quantitative Relationship Between Sugar Intake and Dental Caries: The Need for New Criteria for Developing Goals for Sugar Intake." *BMC Public Health*, September 2014. DOI: 10.1186/1471-2458-14-863. http://bmcpublichealth.biomedcentral.com/articles/10.1186/1471-2458-14-863

Sherwood, Lauralee. *Human Physiology: From Cells to Systems,* Ninth Edition. Independence, KY: Cengage Learning, 2016.

Shibata, S., and N. Suzuki. "Effects of an Indoor Plant on Creative Task performance and Mood." *Scandinavian Journal of Psychology*, 2004; 45: 373–81.

Sifferlin, Alexandra. "Mind Your Reps. Exercise, Especially Weight Lifting, Helps Keep the Brain Sharp." *Time Magazine*, July 16, 2012.

Sifferlin, Alexandra. "Salt Sugar Fat: Q&A with Author Michael Moss." *Time Magazine*, February 26, 2013.

Singh, Gitanjali M., et al. "Estimated Global, Regional, and National Disease Burdens Related to Sugar-Sweetened Beverage Consumption in 2010." American Heart Association, August 25, 2015; 132(8): 639–66. DOI: 10.1161/CIRCULATIONAHA.114.010636. https://www.ncbi.nlm.nih.gov/pmc/articles/PMC4550490/

Smith, Emily Esfahani. "Social Connection Makes a Better Brain." *The Atlantic*, October 29, 2013.

Society for Human Resources Management. "Vacation's Impact on the Workplace Survey." August 22–September 5, 2013. https://www.shrm.org/hr-today/trends-and-forecasting/research-and-surveys/pages/shrm-us-travel-vacation-benefits.aspx

Society for Neuroscience. "Sleep-deprived Brains Alternate Between Normal Activity and 'Power Failure.'" May 2008.

Spain, Erin. "Even Physically Active Women Sit Too Much." October 30, 2012. www.northwestern.edu/newscenter/stories/2012/10/even-physically-active-women-sit-too-much.html

Starfield, B., L. Shi, and J. Macinko. "Contribution of Primary Care to Health Systems and Health." *The Milbank Quarterly*, 2005; 83(3): 457–502.

Starr, Ringo. "Ringo Starr Receives the DLF Lifetime of Peace and Love Award." 2014. http://tmhome.com/experiences/ringo-starr-receives-a-lifetime-award/

Statista. "Statistics and Facts on the Global Business Travel Industry." 2014. http://www.statista.com/topics/2439/global-business-travel-industry/

Steinbeck, John. *Sweet Thursday.* New York: Viking Press, 1954.

Stevens, Richard. "The Key to Feeling Well Rested Isn't Just the Amount of Time You Sleep." *Business Insider*, April 6, 2015.

Stevenson, Robert Louis. *Essay of Travel.* London: Chatto and Windus, 1905.

Stewart, Walter F., et al. "Cost of Lost Productive Work Time among U.S. Workers with Depression." *JAMA*, June 18, 2003; 289(23): 3135–44.

Taris, Toon W. "Investigating the Associations among Overtime Work, Health Behaviors, and Health: A Longitudinal Study among Full-time Employees." *The International Journal of Behavioral Medicine*, 2011; 18: 352–60. DOI: 10.1007/S12529-010-9103-Z

Thaik, Cynthia M. "Take a Vacation for Your Health." *Psychology Today*, May 30, 2013. https://www.psychologytoday.com/blog/the-heart/201305/take-vacation-your-health

The Global Wellness Institute. "Statistics & Facts." www.globalwellnessinstitute.org/statistics-and-facts/

The Notebooks of Leonardo Da Vinci, Complete. Release Date: January 2004 [Ebook #5000], volume 1.

Thomson, J. Arthur. "Vis Medicatrix Naturae." Keynote Address at the Annual Meeting of the British Medical Association, 1914.

Tierney, John. "Do You Suffer from Decision Fatigue?" *New York Times Magazine*, August 17, 2011.

Trichopoulos, Dimitrios. "Siesta in Healthy Adults and Coronary Mortality in the General Population." *Archives of Internal Medicine*, 2007; 167(3): 296–301. DOI: 10.1001/Archinte.167.3.296

Turek, F. W., and P. C. Zee, eds. "The Impact of Changes in Nightlength (Scotoperiod) on Human Sleep." In *Neurobiology of Sleep and Circadian Rhythms* (New York: Marcel Dekker, 1999), 263–85.

Twain, Mark. *The American Claimant*. New York: Charles L. Webster and Company, 1892.

Twain, Mark. *The Innocents Abroad*. Hartford, CT: American Publishing Company, 1869.

Ulrich, Roger S. "View Through a Window May Influence Recovery from Surgery." *Science*, April 27, 1984; 224: 420.

Union of Concerned Scientists. "Added Sugar on the Nutrition Facts Label: Public Comments to the FDA Show Big Food Is Sour on Science." March 2015. http://www.ucsusa.org/center-science-and-democracy/added-sugar-nutrition-facts-label#.vld7y9-rsv4

United States Department of Agriculture. "Meat and Poultry Labeling Terms." August 2015. http://www.fsis.usda.gov/wps/portal/fsis/topics/food-safety-education/get-answers/food-safety-fact-sheets/food-labeling/meat-and-poultry-labeling-terms/meat-and-poultry-labeling-terms

University of Liverpool. "Fish Oil May Stall Effects of Junk Food on Brain." *Science Daily*, May 14, 2013. www.sciencedaily.com/releases/2013/05/130514101455.htm

University of London. "New Study Reveals How Changes in Lifestyle Are Contributing to Dramatic Rise in Obesity." August 28, 2015.

Unterrainer, H. F., et al. "Soul Darkness? Dimensions of Religious/Spiritual Well-Being Among Mood-Disordered Inpatients Compared to Healthy Controls." *Psychopathology*, 2012; 45(5): 310–16. DOI: 10.1159/000336050

US Food & Drug Administration. "Nutritional Labeling and Education Act (NLEA) Requirements (8/94–2/95)." http://www.fda.gov/iceci/inspections/inspectionguides/ucm074948.htm

US Travel Association. "Travel Effect Report." 2013.

US Travel Association. "US Travel Answer Sheet." 2015. https://www.ustravel.org/sites /default/files/media%20root/document/us_travel_answersheet_dec2015_final%20 (2).pdf

Van Dijk, Sheri. *Calming the Emotional Store: Using Dialectical Behavior Therapy Skills to Manage Your Emotions and Balance Your Life*. Oakland, CA: New Harbinger Publications, 2012.

Variety Power of Women Event, 2013. https://www.youtube.com/watch?v =G4Q0oX8wquU

Vaze, K. M., and V. K. Sharma. "On the Adaptive Significance of Circadian Clocks for Their Owners." *Chronobiology International*, May 2013; 30(4): 413–33. DOI: 10.3100/07420528.2012.754457. Epub March 4, 2013.

Vickery, Donald, Larry Matson, and Carol Vickery. *Live Young, Think Young, Be Young*. Boulder, CO: Bull Publishing Company, 2012.

Walker, Rob. "Jeff Bezos, Amazon.Com, Because 'Optimism Is Essential.'" *Inc. Magazine*, 2004. http://www.inc.com/magazine/20040401/25bezos.html

Wang, Q., et al. "Voluntary Exercise Counteracts Aβ25-35-induced Memory Impairment in Mice." *Behavioural Brain Research*, 2013; 256. DOI: 10.1016/J.Bbr.2013.09.024. http://www.sciencedirect.com/science/article/pii/S0166432813005743

Ward Thompson, C., J. Roe, P. Aspinall, R. Mitchell, A. Clow, and D. Miller. "More Green Space Is Linked to Less Stress in Deprived Communities: Evidence from Salivary Cortisol Patterns." *Landscape and Urban Planning*, 2012; 105: 221–29.

Weekes, John. "Mediterranean Diet Could Help Men With Prostate Cancer." *New Zealand Herald*, July 22, 2015.

Weil, Andrew. *Natural Health, Natural Medicine*. Boston: Houghton Mifflin Company, 2004.

Weil, Andrew. "Vitamin Library." www.drweil.com/drw/u/pag00321/vitamin-library-supplement-facts.html

Weil, Andrew. "Integrative Medicine: A Vital Part of the New Health Care System." Testimony Before the Committee on Health, Education, Labor, and Pensions, United States Senate, February 26, 2009.

Weir, Kirsten. "The Exercise Effect," *American Psychological Association*, December 2011; 42(11). http://www.apa.org/monitor/2011/12/exercise.aspx

Westman, M., and D. Etzion. "The Impact of Vacation and Job Stress on Burnout and Absenteeism." *Psychology and Health*, 2001; 16(5): 595–606.

Wheeler, Mark. "How to Build a Bigger Brain." *UCLA Newsroom*, May 12, 2009.

Wheeler, Mark. "Evidence Builds that Meditation Strengthens the Brain, UCLA Researchers Say." *UCLA Newsroom*, March 14, 2012.

Woolf, Virginia. *A Room of One's Own*. London: Hogarth Press, 1929.

World Bank Statistic. http://data.worldbank.org/indicator/SP.DYN.LE00.IN

World Health Organization. "Global Status Report on Non-Communicable Diseases Chapter 5: Improving Health Care: Individual Interventions." 1998. http://www.who. int/nmh/publications/ncd_report_chapter5.pdf

World Health Organization. "Q&A on Artemisinin Resistance." February 2015. http://who.int/malaria/media/artemisinin_resistance_qa/en/

World Health Organization. "Wellness." http://www.who.int/about/definition/en/print.html

World Health Organization. "WHO Calls on Countries to Reduce Sugars Intake among Adults and Children." March 4, 2015. www.who.int/mediacentre/news/releases/2015/sugar-guideline/en/

Wright, H. R. "Effect of Light Wavelength on Suppression and Phase Delay of the Melatonin Rhythm." *Chronobiology International*, September 2001; 18(5): 801–8.

Wu, A. J. "Dietary Omega-3 Fatty Acids Normalize BDNF Levels, Reduce Oxidative Damage, and Counteract Learning Disability after Traumatic Brain Injury in Rats." *Neurotrauma*, October 2004; 21(10): 1457–67.

Xie, L., et al. "Sleep Initiated Fluid Flux Drives Metabolite Clearance from the Adult Brain." *Science*, October 18, 2013. DOI: 10.1126/Science.1241224

Yamamoto, T., et al. "Effect of Sauna Bathing and Beer Ingestion on Plasma Concentrations of Purine Bases." *Metabolism*, June 2004; 53(6): 772–76.

Yang, Quanhe. "Morbidity and Mortality Weekly Report (MMWR), Center for Disease Control, Vital Signs: Predicted Heart Age and Racial Disparities in Heart Age among U.S. Adults at the State Level." September 1, 2015.

Yang, Q. "Added Sugar Intake and Cardiovascular Diseases Mortality among US Adults." *JAMA Internal Medicine*, April 2014; 174(4): 516–24. DOI: 10.1001/Jamainternmed.2013.13563

Yesawich, Peter C. "National Travel Monitor: Travelers Trading Down, Not Out." *Hotel & Motel Management*, January 9, 2009; 224(10): 20.

Young, Richard and Jennifer DeVoe. "Who Will Have Health Insurance in the Future? An Updated Projection." *Annals of Family Medicine*, 2012; 10: 156–62. DOI: 10.1370/afm.1348

Yue, Pengying. "Neck/Shoulder Pain and Low Back Pain among School Teachers in China, Prevalence and Risk Factors." *BMC Public Health*, 2012; 12: 789. DOI: 10.1186/1471-2458-12-789

Zevon, Warren. "I'll Sleep When I'm Dead." *Warren Zevon*. Asylum Records, 1976.

Zimmermann, Julia and Franz J. Neyer. "Do We Become a Different Person When Hitting the Road? Personality Development of Sojourners." *Journal of Personality and Social Psychology*, September 2013; 105(3): 515–30. http://psycnet.apa.org/?&fa=main.doilanding&doi=10.1037/a0033019

INDEX

ABOUT THE AUTHOR

Linden Schaffer is a wellness travel expert, consultant, and the founder of Pravassa, the first wellness travel company. Since founding Pravassa in 2009, Linden has been leading travelers around the world on wellness tours, which offer group and individualized itineraries for the people and companies that are looking to restore productivity and creativity. As a winner of the prestigious British Airways Face of Opportunity contest, Linden contributes to columns in *The Huffington Post* and *mindbodygreen*, is a regular speaker at conferences around the country, and has participated in international conferences in Colombia, India, and Spain in order to bring wellness travel opportunities to these countries. When Linden is not traveling the world, she is based in New York City.